Healing Holidays: Itinerant Patients, Therapeutic Locales and the Quest for Health

This volume on medical tourism includes contributions by anthropologists and historians on a variety of health-seeking modes of travel and leisure. It brings together analyses of recent trends of 'medical tourism', such as underinsured middle-class Americans travelling to India for surgery, pious Middle Eastern couples seeking assisted reproduction outside their borders, or consumers of the exotic in search of alternative healing, with analyses of the centuries-old Euro-American tradition of travelling to spas. Rather than seeing these two forms of medical travel as being disparate, the book demonstrates that, as noted in the introduction "what makes patients itinerant in both the old and new kind of medical travel is either a perceived shortage or constraint at 'home', or the sense of having reached a particular kind of therapeutic impasse, with the two often so intertwined that it is difficult to tell them apart. The constraint may stem from things as diverse as religious injunctions, legal hurdles, social approbation, or seasonal affliction; and the shortage can range from a lack of privacy, of insurance, technology, competence, or enough therapeutic resources that can address issues and conditions that patients have. If these two intertwined strands are responsible for most medical tourism, then which locales seem to have therapeutic resources are those that are either 'natural,' in the form of water or climate; legal, in the form of a culture that does not stigmatise patients; or technological and professional, in the form of tests, equipment, or expertise, unavailable or affordable at home; or in the form of novel therapeutic possibilities that promise to resolve irresolvable issues".

This book was originally published as a special issue of *Anthropology & Medicine*.

Harish Naraindas is Associate Professor at Jawaharlal Nehru University, India, Adjunct Associate Professor at the University of Iowa, USA, and was Joint-appointments Professor (2008–12), South Asia Institute, University of Heidelberg, Germany. His latest publication is the co-edited book, *Asymmetrical Conversations: Contestations, Circumventions and the Blurring of Therapeutic Boundaries* (2014).

Cristiana Bastos is Senior Research Fellow at the Institute of Social Sciences, University of Lisbon, Portugal, she has held visiting professorships at Brown and UMass Dartmouth, USA, and authored books and articles on health, science, colonial medicine, migration, displacement; her upcoming volumes are on Goa and on race and migration in early twentieth century USA.

Healing Holidays: Itinerant Patients, Therapeutic Locales and the Quest for Health

Edited by
Harish Naraindas and Cristiana Bastos

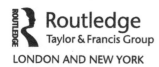

Routledge
Taylor & Francis Group

LONDON AND NEW YORK

First published 2015 by Routledge

2 Park Square, Milton Park, Abingdon, Oxon, OX14 4RN
605 Third Avenue, New York, NY 10017

Routledge is an imprint of the Taylor & Francis Group, an informa business

First issued in paperback 2020

British Library Cataloguing in Publication Data
A catalogue record for this book is available from the British Library

ISBN 13: 978-1-138-80665-8 (hbk)
ISBN 13: 978-0-367-73913-3 (pbk)

Typeset in Times New Roman
by RefineCatch Limited, Bungay, Suffolk

Publisher's Note
The publisher accepts responsibility for any inconsistencies that may have
arisen during the conversion of this book from journal articles to book chapters,
namely the possible inclusion of journal terminology.

Disclaimer
Every effort has been made to contact copyright holders for their permission to
reprint material in this book. The publishers would be grateful to hear from any
copyright holder who is not here acknowledged and will undertake to rectify
any errors or omissions in future editions of this book.

Contents

Citation Information

The chapters in this book were originally published in *Anthropology & Medicine*, volume 18, issue 1 (April 2011). When citing this material, please use the original page numbering for each article, as follows:

Chapter 1
Introduction: Special Issue for Anthropology & Medicine: Healing Holidays? Itinerant patients, therapeutic locales and the quest for health
Harish Naraindas and Cristiana Bastos
Anthropology & Medicine, volume 18, issue 1 (April 2011) pp. 1–6

Chapter 2
Taking the (southern) waters: science, slavery, and nationalism at the Virginia springs
Lauren E. LaFauci
Anthropology & Medicine, volume 18, issue 1 (April 2011) pp. 7–22

Chapter 3
Seeking 'energy' vs. pain relief in spas in Brazil (Caldas da Imperatriz) and Portugal (Termas da Sulfúrea)
Maria Manuel Quintela
Anthropology & Medicine, volume 18, issue 1 (April 2011) pp. 23–35

Chapter 4
From sulphur to perfume: spa and SPA at Monchique, Algarve
Cristiana Bastos
Anthropology & Medicine, volume 18, issue 1 (April 2011) pp. 37–53

Chapter 5
Health tourism in a Czech health spa
Amy R. Speier
Anthropology & Medicine, volume 18, issue 1 (April 2011) pp. 55–66

Chapter 6
Of relics, body parts and laser beams: the German Heilpraktiker and his Ayurvedic spa
Harish Naraindas
Anthropology & Medicine, volume 18, issue 1 (April 2011) pp. 67–86

Chapter 7
Globalization and gametes: reproductive 'tourism,' Islamic bioethics, and Middle Eastern modernity
Marcia C. Inhorn
Anthropology & Medicine, volume 18, issue 1 (April 2011) pp. 87–103

Chapter 8
Affective journeys: the emotional structuring of medical tourism in India
Harris Solomon
Anthropology & Medicine, volume 18, issue 1 (April 2011) pp. 105–118

Chapter 9
Selling medical travel to US patient-consumers: the cultural appeal of website marketing messages
Elisa J. Sobo, Elizabeth Herlihy and Mary Bicker
Anthropology & Medicine, volume 18, issue 1 (April 2011) pp. 119–136

Chapter 10
Afterword: Historical reflections on medical travel
George Weisz
Anthropology & Medicine, volume 18, issue 1 (April 2011) pp. 137–144

Please direct any queries you may have about the citations to
clsuk.permissions@cengage.com

INTRODUCTION

Healing holidays? Itinerant patients, therapeutic locales and the quest for health

Harish Naraindas[a] and Cristiana Bastos[b]

[a]*Jawaharlal Nehru University, India;* [b]*Social Sciences Institute, University of Lisbon, Portugal*

This special issue on medical 'tourism' draws upon the panel 'Healing Holidays' held at the Society for Medical Anthropology's 50th anniversary conference in 2009. The issue brings together anthropologists and historians whose work addresses the historical evolution and contemporary transformation of the traditional spa built around the iconic image of 'taking the waters', and the more recent phenomenon of medical 'tourism', with its super-speciality hospitals and clinics that repair and replace organs and body parts, or assist infertile people in their quest for conception. The final article addresses medical travel websites that serve as mediators between patients and their destinations in their itinerant quest for health.

The articles as a whole problematise whether holidays can be healing and whether healing can be a holiday, exemplified by the often-raised question of whether the spa is medicine or vacation. Using different perspectives and ethnographic contexts, the first five articles address the spa – which in the contemporary imagination is associated with a pleasurable vacation with some health thrown in, best described by the currently popular word 'wellness'. Partly fashioned by literary and cinematic conventions, this picture of the spa is often used as a form of social commentary on the contemporary middle class. In earlier eras, it was used in much the same way to comment on the aristocracy and the rising bourgeoisie. Or, as is the case in the opening article, spas could be used in the mid-nineteenth century America to craft a distinctly southern ideology of race identity. This function has its counterparts in the spas of the colonial tropics (Jennings 2006) and continental Europe. While this vein of using the spa as a form of social commentary runs through all the articles in this issue, these papers also, and in fundamental ways, point to the fact that until recently in the Euro-American world, the spa lay within the provenance of conventional medicine. This is still the case on the European continent, where the traditional training in medical hydrology, balneology, and climatology available in formal curricula evolved into the specialty of spa medicine. Although not everyone in the medical profession in Europe endorse its 'scientificity', spa medicine (or 'thermalism') is a legitimate practice in the continent.

The opening piece by LaFauci fuses these two strands – of reading the spa as social commentary and investigating it as a site of medical practice – by showing that the constructed distinctiveness of the southern waters of Virginia is clearly located within the medical lexicon of the time, allowing white Southerners to see them and use them as a cure to a southern climate and its southern diseases, reinforcing, with this difference, a distinct southern ideology of nationalism.

Hence, not only was the spa once legitimate medicine in the Euro-American world, but it continues to be so on the European continent, where it is supervised and supported by the state and is a reimbursable medical expense to varying degrees in the different countries, although this is now dwindling. This situation is a far cry from its practice in either contemporary America or Brazil, where the spa as medicine slowly fizzled out from the early part of the twentieth century, reappearing instead as an alternative healing practice.

Climatology and medical hydrology developed a body of knowledge about the healing properties of locales, with their special composition of airs and waters. Within these disciplines, mineral waters were at times considered medicinal substances capable of curing patients of long-standing chronic conditions, or at least relieving their worst symptoms. The uses of waters for healing and for leisure had been around for thousands of years, often supported by religious beliefs and rituals, which medicine came either to prolong or to replace. The developments of medical hydrology helped classify the different therapeutic locales according to the diseases and conditions that they were best thought to cure. And to *cure* was what many patients were looking for at the different spas; and unlike today's image of the spa as a site only for the posh and well-heeled, there were many poor and indigent patients taking the waters, as shown by Brockliss (1990), Mackaman (1998), and Weisz (2001) for France, and Bastos (this issue) for Portugal.

This double argument of the spa as medicine and the spa as a place that also catered to the hoi polloi re-appears across the articles. In Virginia, one can see, through the *mise-en-scene* that LaFauci creates, that despite the erasing of enslaved black people from the narrative of the spa – in which at best they appear as servants with separate quarters and different fees – there was also a 'black sulphur spring' set apart at one of the most prominent resorts, and in others, where enslaved people could be treated for various illnesses in exchange for their labour. In Europe, through the *Termas* in Portugal, or the Czech Marienska Lanske, or the Ayurvedic spa in Germany, one can see that the spa is the site of salvation for patients with rheumatic pains, unresolved and painful chronic diseases, and kidney stones. Additionally, in a place like Marienbad, until the collapse of communism, the spa was both a reward for hard work and was part of an economic rationale of extending the productive life of the worker.

Such a double rationale, supported by state socialism in the former Czechoslovakia and by a kind of socialised insurance scheme in the former West Germany, seems to symbolise the democratisation of a set of therapeutic and social practices that were once seen to be the sole preserve of the aristocracy and the bourgeoisie. While it is evident from the early history of Monchique, Portugal, that this state of things is partly an illusion, the argument is not untrue, as even those places that were indeed the sole provenance of the elites are now opened to other social classes, enabled by state support and by various models of health insurance.

The continental European spa, caught in a web of science, medicine, and socialised insurance, emerges slowly in the early twentieth century and fully consolidates itself by the mid 1970s. But with the collapse of state socialism in the East, and the shrinking of the welfare state in the West, the spa was re-invented as a wellness destination, leading to tensions and conflicts (as in Marienbad), or at times to creative pluralism (as in Monchique), or setting out in wholly new directions (as in Germany). While Bastos and Speier show this transformation with respect to Portugal and Czechoslovakia/Czech Republic, Quintela's comparative study of Brazil and Portugal shows how this change is, in part, a replay of a phenomenon that occurred in Brazil in the 1920s. Here, the older medical spa, as it steps out of the realms of both conventional medicine and state support, reinvents itself as alternative therapy and a wellness destination, where a focus on energising the body – rather than pain and its alleviation – becomes the new idiom through which bodies are made whole and healthy. In Monchique, by contrast, this replay creatively combines the old and new. Rather than jettisoning the medical aspects of the spa, it offers patients a variety and choice of treatment not envisaged in the old spa, thus lifting the sagging spa economy – already hit by shrinking social insurance and a reduced, ageing clientele – and making it into a trendy consumer product. In Marienbad, on the other hand, the collapse of socialism sees the exit of the trade unions and workers, and with them, Czech patients more generally. These spas now begin to compete for wealthy German spa goers, and for a new group of English-speaking tourists from the UK and North America, who, unlike the Germans, are not familiar with the conventional spa etiquette and its rituals. This confluence of tourists leads to tensions and contradictions between the old notion of the spa and the new vacationer in search of pleasurable relaxation.

These transformations and the ensuing contradictions are played out on a grand scale in Germany, the largest spa-going nation in Europe, where the spa is captured in the three German terms of *Bad* (bath), *Therme*, (a hot mineral water source or pool), and the *Kur* (cure, or the regimen). It is evident from the German case that the *Kur-Bad* or the *Therme* slowly re-invents itself by expanding its therapeutic repertoire. This re-invention, in response to a shrinking insurance fund and an ageing and unproductive population (which is true for the whole of Europe), leads the large *Kur* industry to look at new therapeutic formats like Ayurveda, which is now appropriated and organised as a *Kur* experience with its own *Kur* regimen, although it is removed from the *Therme* or the *Bad*. This is enabled in part by the German ability to accommodate therapeutic pluralism and attention to order, best exemplified in the institution of the *Heilpraktiker* or 'lay healer', who is allowed to practice, with some kind of nominal training, a host of therapies. This kind of rule-bound, licensed, poly-therapeutics, enshrined in a non-university trained non-physician, and the surprising mimicking of this kind of poly-therapeutics by university-trained physicians, provides the larger climate within which the *Kur* readily transforms itself into new therapeutic formats, while the new formats are minted in the idiom of the *Kur*.

While German therapeutic practice exemplifies the blurring of boundaries between what is seen as a contrast between the spa and medicine in the non-European world, this blurring of boundaries is equally evident in all the articles dealing with the spa in the western world, past and present. Thus, a 'healing holiday' is not a contradiction in terms, as one would read from contemporary conventions that establish that people should be cured (and not healed) by hospitalisation or by the ubiquitous pill. Healing and pleasure can indeed coexist well, albeit in tension; travelling to posh locales for medical reasons may raise judgments and comments about the nature of that healing, counter-argued by an emphasis on the harshness of the spa regimen. The current transformations of the European spa, where 'patients' seem to turn into 'consumers', and 'cures' turn into 'commodities', best exemplified by the experiences at Monchique and Marienbad, may enhance the distance between the pleasurable and the painful sides of the experience. Hence, it is not surprising that in Germany the word *Kur* was officially erased from the lexicon in 2000, although it survives in popular vernacular: its survival is due in part to inertia and in part to a perceived need for it, which is explored in richly textured ways by both Quintela in Brazil and Naraindas in Germany.

It is in the light of this orthodox norm of organic pathology requiring expensive hospitalisation, which is increasingly beyond the reach of uninsured and under-insured patients in the first world, that the second proposition of healing-as-holiday has run into most difficulty. This new kind of travel, often for surgical procedures, is even harder to reconcile with a holiday than the spa regimen that often included pleasurable pursuits. This has, understandably enough, led authors to either discard the term (Inhorn, this issue), or call it 'medical travel' (Sobo 2009, and this issue), or even suggest that such patients are in a kind of exile (Inhorn and Patrizio 2009).

'Medical exile' is best exemplified in this issue by Inhorn's moving depiction of a rural and well-to-do Sunni Islamic couple's quest for conception. In contrast to the stereotypical picture of Islamic societies as blithely polygamous, where the stigma of infertility is believed to result in the man taking another wife, a not-so-young couple, after close to two decades of marriage, repeatedly set out to conceive. Disallowed by Sunni law to have donor eggs, the couple goes in search of Shia gametes. Since any kind of surrogacy is frowned upon, their travel is conducted under the guise of a holiday. Here, the holiday functions as a trope for a painful and traumatic quest, relieved in this case by a deep and abiding love that unites the couple, who are simultaneously surrounded by a horde of children produced by the man's several siblings. What Inhorn calls a 'reproscape,' this kind of 'holiday-exile' is propelled by legal and religious injunctions, associated with technology and money, and concerned at every moment with movements and boundary crossings between Sunni and Shia bodies and American gametes in Arab wombs.

If affect is easily but implicitly at the centre of this holiday-exile narrative, in the case of Harris Solomon's depiction of Euro-American travel to India, affect is explicitly at the centre of his narrative. Solomon argues that emotion, rather than being ancillary to any analysis of medical travel, should be explicitly addressed as conditioning medical travel. Drawing on a body of theoretical literature that has attempted to address this through the notions of 'emotional economy' or 'affective economy', he uses *affect* as both a thematic and theoretical resource to show how emotion is central to the selling of medical tourism by five-star Indian hospitals to prospective Euro-American clients. He sees affect as 'the linchpin between everyday sentiments and objects, clinical care, and medical travel's institutional structuring'. It can appear in many forms, including, for example, as fully accredited, high-quality, and worry-free care for anxious and prospective patients. In Solomon's narrative, this is best embodied by a personal and exclusive attendant, who soothes the passage of a nervous American couple into an Indian landscape of sights and smells that assault their senses. While the couple is driven into exile by high cost and no insurance, an Englishman is cast into exile by an insensitive and uncaring National Health Service (NHS), which refuses to give him an MRI for his lower back pain as it has decided that his pain is in 'his head' (imaginary) and not in his spine. This lack of affect at home, which should be seen as a fusion of the emotional, the economic and the medical, is offset by the abundance of affect at the Icon Indian hospital, with its fawning nurses and personal attendants, and with the continuous crooning of care beamed over its in-house television. The acme of this care bubble is the immediate MRI on arrival, which results in a quick diagnosis of his problem, which the NHS had missed over 20 years, and subsequent surgery that resolves the pain.

The same affect, through the central and recurring trope of a 'worry-free experience', is sold by Medical Travel Agencies' websites to prospective American patients. Through a novel and carefully conceived method, Elisa Sobo presents an ethnographic account of American MTA websites to show how a particular picture of the patient as a savvy consumer is constructed. This consumer, who knows what is best by consulting an array of information before exercising her choice, is also a patient who will be fully attended to by various kinds of concierge services in a world-class facility and operated upon by world-class (read: American-trained) doctors. Sobo shows how these savvy consumers exercising choice are at odds with the cognate construction of patients who want to be fully looked after. But the MTA websites resolve this contradiction by presenting these two facets in different parts of their sites; in the process, they iron out – if not altogether negate – possible contradictions into experiences that at once promise to be self-fashioned and a worry-free travel bubble.

It is evident that what makes patients itinerant in both the old and new kind of medical travel is either a perceived shortage or constraint at 'home', or the sense of having reached a particular kind of therapeutic impasse, with the two often so intertwined that it is difficult to tell them apart. The constraint may stem from things as diverse as religious injunctions, legal hurdles, social approbation, or seasonal affliction; and the shortage can range from a lack of privacy, of insurance, technology, competence, or enough therapeutic resources that can address issues and conditions that patients have.

While those constraints and shortages may be an amalgam of the legal, social, religious and technological, and may be directly responsible for unresolved health issues, they are also due to a therapeutic impasse resulting from orthodox medicine's inability to provide a solution for many patients' problems. If these two intertwined strands are responsible for most medical tourism, then which locales seem to have therapeutic resources are those that are either 'natural,' in the form of water or climate; legal, in the form of a culture that does not stigmatise patients; or technological and professional, in the form of tests, equipment, or expertise, unavailable or affordable at home; or in the form of novel therapeutic possibilities that promise to resolve irresolvable issues.

What is on offer by way of this short introduction is only a kind of scaffolding for the articles in this issue. Each of them addresses not only the issues above but several others; and they all do so by bringing their own theoretical perspectives to bear upon their respective problems. The readers are invited to journey with them, in an attempt to understand better why patients travel to particular locales in their quest for health.

References

Brockliss, L.W. 1990. The development of the spa in seventeenth-century France. *Medical History Supplement*, no. 10: 23–47.

Inhorn, M., and P. Patrizio. 2009. Rethinking reproductive 'tourism' as reproductive 'exile'. *Fertility and Sterility* 29, no. 3: 904–6.

Jennings, Eric T. 2006. *Curing the colonizers: Hydrotherapy, climatology, and French colonial spas*. Durham: Duke University Press.

Mackaman, Douglas Peter. 1998. *Leisure settings: Bourgeois culture, medicine, and the spa in modern France*. Chicago: University of Chicago Press.

Sobo, E.J. 2009. Medical travel: What it means and why it matters. *Medical Anthropology* 29, no. 1: 326–35.

Weisz, George. 2001. Spas, mineral waters and hydrological science in twentieth-century France. *Isis* 92, no. 3: 451–83.

Taking the (southern) waters: science, slavery, and nationalism at the Virginia springs

Lauren E. LaFauci

English Department, Simpson College, Indianola, Iowa, USA

'Taking the (southern) waters' argues that, in the pre-Civil War period, the space of Virginia's mineral water resorts and the philosophy of southern hydropathic medicine enabled – indeed, fostered – white southerners' constructions of a 'nationalist,' proslavery ideology. In the first half of the paper, the author explains how white southern health-seekers came to view the springs region as a medicinal resource peculiarly designed for the healing of southern diseases and for the restoration of white southern constitutions; in the second half, she shows how physical and social aspects of the resorts, such as architectural choices and political events, supported and encouraged proslavery ideologies. Taken together, these medical-social analyses reveal how elite white southerners in the antebellum period came to associate the health of their peculiarly 'southern' bodies with the future health of an independent southern nation, one that elided black bodily presence at the same time that its social structures and scientific apparatuses relied upon enslaved black labor.

In 1851, as sectional tensions between the northern and southern regions of the United States intensified, physician and author William Burke began to imagine the mineral waters of Virginia as a site of national healing, as a location for the restoration of severed ties between the two regions:

> And to the people of the North, and to those of the South, the *capillaries* of the Union, I would say, flow on through your respective conduits, to the social heart of the mother of states – Old Virginia. If your streams have been rendered turbid by prejudice; if too much carbonic acid, or unwholesome bile has mingled in their currents; she will urge you on to the healthy lungs in her parental bosom; she will oxygenize your *ill-blood* in the pure atmosphere of her mountains; she will render it ruddy and healthy, and send it back bounding with impulse, inspiring fraternal affections and sympathies, and connecting the frame of our social and political Union by tissues that shall not decay, and ligaments that can never be loosened. (Burke 1851, 293, emphasis in original)

In his nostalgic reference to 'Old Virginia' as the 'mother of states,' Burke not only reminds his northern and southern readers of their common colonial and republican origins, but he also constructs Virginia as the healthful (female) body of the nation to which its children must return in order to (re)gain health. In his construction,

Virginia possesses 'healthy lungs in her parental bosom' and a 'pure atmosphere' in her mountains; both of these physical elements transform the 'children,' the people of the North and South, from ill to blooming health. In turn, this restoration of healthfulness would suffice for restoring socio-political relations: physical health is apparently all that the two sections need in order to reconcile their difficulties. That is, Burke suggests that the problems between the North and the South are a kind of short-term malady, a seasonal malaise, that requires but a short stay in a salutary climate – in the genteel space of the springs – before all might be forgiven. The violent troubles between the two 'siblings' are not a systemic cancer, or even a fatal intermittent fever, but rather an imbalance of bile, an excess of carbonic acid, a dearth of oxygen.

Although Burke penned four separate editions of *The mineral springs of Virginia*, under slightly different titles, in 1842, 1846, 1851, and 1853, the passage above first appears in the 1851 edition. Thus, between 1842 and 1851, Burke apparently began to think about Virginia, particularly the spaces of the Virginia springs, as a symbolic 'ligament' between North and South, a 'connecting frame of our social and political Union.' A number of events transpired during this interlude that might have motivated Burke to call for a restoration of 'fraternal affections and sympathies' between North and South, including the vast expansion of the territory of the United States following the Treaty of Guadalupe Hidalgo that ended the US–Mexican War, the rush to California for the mining of gold, the election of two Whig presidents (Zachary Taylor and Millard Fillmore), and, perhaps most influential to Burke's words, the passage of the Compromise of 1850. Henry Clay's Compromise managed to gall both southerners and northerners, precipitating a new era of heated sectionalism as Americans of all political stripes, in all states and territories, were required to abide by the Fugitive Slave Law. The 1850s would see further escalating conflicts before Abraham Lincoln's election in 1860 precipitated the secession of the southern states.

Burke's solution to the increasing sectional strife is an environmental one: just breathe Virginia's pure mountain air, he says, and spend time remembering our common origins, and you will feel renewed affection and sympathy toward us. Speaking as a southerner to an imagined (and embittered) national audience, he mobilizes the historical antecedent of the Old Dominion legacy and a presentist geographical-medical exceptionality in order to urge his readers to visit the springs. In his anthropomorphic construction of Virginia as a healing mother to which both sections of the nation must return in order to get well, Burke suggests that the health of the nation is measured by the strength of its social bonds and its political unity.[1]

While Burke optimistically urges residents of the North and South to reunite in the springs region of Virginia, most archival evidence suggests that the spaces of the springs did not attract visitors from the North in great droves, especially at the late date of 1851. The predominantly white and southern visitors to the resorts certainly did adopt his assertion of Virginia's healing capacities, but they did so not to promote reconciliation between the two sections, but rather to bolster southern unity and nationalism. As North and South migrated further apart, white southerners at the springs represented Virginia's mineral waters as especially adapted for the 'peculiar' diseases plaguing the South and for the 'peculiar' constitution of the southern body. White southerners in the antebellum period thus came to view Virginia's mineral springs as a peculiarly southern natural resource, one that revealed both the distinctiveness of their own southern bodies and the 'naturalness' of southern waters for curing their ailments. Just as Burke connected social and political health with national health, so too did white southerners at the Virginia springs – though to opposing ends: in linking the physical healing of their southern bodies with the curative powers of Virginia mineral waters, wealthy white elites employed the medicinal resources of the springs as an index of the future strength of an independent southern nation.

To show how the mineral waters of the South helped white southerners construct an ideology of independence, this essay first explains how these valetudinarians came to conceive of the springs region as a veritable pharmacopeia of watery resources designed to alleviate peculiarly southern diseases and to restore peculiarly southern constitutions. The second half of the essay shows how the local spaces of the springs propped up southern proslavery ideologies through their architectural choices, social customs, and political staging. While visitors to the springs primarily viewed the resorts as salutary aids, their curative experiences there – undertaken with other southern white elites – served to consolidate their collective proslavery ideologies at the same time they restored individual bodily health. As visitors from across the southern states came to identify 'the springs' with 'the South,' they also came to identify themselves as adherents to a common ideology that was simultaneously local and national in scope. And because that shared experience took place at the healing fountain of 'Old Virginia,' white southerners associated the health of their bodies with the future health of their burgeoning nation.

Peculiar adaptations: southern waters, southern bodies

Using water to cure disease or alleviate pain was neither unique to the North American continent nor to nineteenth-century medical practice. The Greek physician Hippocrates prescribed water for illness, and hydropathy accorded well with Galenic humoral theory, which strongly influenced seventeenth- and eighteenth-century medicine in Europe and in the American colonies. Because medical therapeutics during this period relied to a great extent on the bleeding, purging, and general evacuating of offending substances, physicians and laypeople alike encouraged the use of water for bathing, which they believed permeated the body and improved the internal balance of fluids. Both colonials and Native Americans in North America had looked to mineral and thermal springs for improved health: American Indians on the eastern seaboard – and, as white settlers would later learn, in the mountain West – used mineral and thermal springs in religious ceremonies, and they revered many individual springs as sacred (Shalinsky 1985, 40–1). In the late seventeenth century, Anglo-Americans in northeastern cities visited Lynn Red Springs (near Boston) and Yellow Springs (near Philadelphia). By the mid-eighteenth century, early colonials were visiting some of the larger and more abundant springs in Virginia, including Berkeley Springs, Warm Springs, and Hot Springs. George Washington visited Berkeley Springs[2] in March 1748 and returned with his wife and stepdaughter several times in the 1760s. By the 1770s, an estimated 2000 visitors enjoyed the springs of Virginia in the high season of July and August alone, and this demand for access led colonial leaders in Williamsburg to collect £900 in order to construct a 'good Coach-Road' over the mountains to the springs in Augusta County (Bridenbaugh 1946, 163–4).

Virginians were not the only ones to recognize the value of their mineral waters to bodily health: South Carolina's low-country planters had by the late eighteenth century come to view their own rural residences as 'unsafe' in the summer months, which initiated an annual migration of white South Carolinians to the mountainous Virginia springs region throughout the 'sickly season' (Brewster 1947, 7–8). Thus, by the time Thomas Jefferson catalogued the state's medicinal springs in his *Notes on the State of Virginia* (Jefferson 1999, 36–8), the mineral waters of Virginia were fast gaining ground as a valuable 'native' southern resource.

Elite whites across the southeastern states came in the first decades of the nineteenth century to view the annual summer trip to the springs as absolutely necessary to the maintenance of health and the prevention of disease at home. Escaping the yellow fever that often plagued urban port cities or the localized cholera epidemics that swept rural farms, these white slave owners flocked to the Virginia springs region from early May to late October or early November, when the danger of contracting seasonal diseases had largely passed.[3] As cultural historians of the region have pointed out,[4] both healthy white southerners and 'invalids' sought health and strength there, and both healthy and sick sojourners believed that the mineral and thermal waters would provide strength and sustenance to all bodies that had been weakened by residence in a warm southern climate, whether black or white, sick or healthy.

Taking the waters became so popular among white southerners that when the first shots were fired at Fort Sumter in April 1861, those in search of health or leisure had no fewer than 32 different mineral water resorts to choose from in Virginia alone.[5] Encompassing an area of about 110 miles in parts of today's West Virginia and Virginia, the chain of resorts dotting the Allegany and Blue Ridge Mountains in the 'springs region' included the Berkeley, Hot, Red Sulphur, Salt Sulphur, Sweet, Warm, and White Sulphur Springs, some of the oldest and most established health resorts in the nation. As taking the waters became a more popular form of treatment for various illnesses, other springs emerged, such as the All Healing, Alleghany, Bath Alum, Buffalo Lithia, Capon, Dibrell's, Fauquier White Sulphur, Gray Sulphur, Montgomery White Sulphur, Orrick's Sulphur, Rawley's, Red Sweet, Roanoke Red Sulphur, Shannondale, Stribling's, Warrenton, and Yellow Sulphur Springs. By the mid-nineteenth century, all of these springs would have been well known to physicians and lay people alike, not just as abstract geographical locations or as places for relaxation and recreation, but as specific medicinal springs adapted to specific ailments.

That white southerners imagined the Virginia springs in this way – as medical resources with 'peculiar' strengths for particular diseases – constituted a divergence from the views of their contemporaries in the northern states. In places like Saratoga Springs, New York, or Brattleboro, Vermont, the 'water cure' comprised one single part of a suite of lifestyle changes designed to promote individual wellness. Led by health reformers Joel Shew, Russell Trall, Mary Gove Nichols, and Thomas Nichols, northern hydropathy exploded between 1840 and 1890, with the founding of over 200 sanatoriums, several professional journals, and a handful of therapeutic institutions geared toward educating the next generation of hydropathic medical practitioners. This hydropathic culture incorporated (and was incorporated by) a number of hygienic and societal reform efforts, including the anti-slavery, anti-tobacco, dress reform, temperance, and vegetarian movements. These broader societal and health concerns of the northern hydropathists stemmed from their widespread dis-ease with contemporary United States culture, and they believed that large-scale societal reform could be achieved through encouraging a healthy citizenry (Cayleff 1988, 83; Green 1986, 17).[6] Thus, for northern health-seekers and water-cure practitioners, a stay at the springs was a way of life rather than a crisis intervention (Cayleff 1988, 84, 89) – that is, patients took the waters not because they were dangerously ill, but because they desired a more healthy way of living. This philosophy – that 'right living' and good health went hand-in-hand – meant that northern hydropathists argued that disease was rooted in the individual, not in the environment: ill health resulted from one's actions, whether in eating, sleeping, drinking, or exercising, and not from the land, climate, or air-borne miasms.

The reality of southern epidemics and of a general constitutional malaise during the 'sickly season' meant that southerners, whether sick or well, early learned not to attribute the cause of illness to individuals, but rather to the environment around them. Of course, they agreed with their northern counterparts that diet and 'constitution' played a role in one's susceptibility to illness, but most southerners rooted the causes of diseases in the air, climate, or environment more broadly rather than in the moral or physical failings of themselves. Because they believed a malicious southern nature to be the primary source of their illness, white southerners came to value the springs region precisely for its beneficent, healthful environment – particularly its climate, its pure mountain air, and its proximity to 'wild' nature – and for its status as a medicinal natural resource, a veritable pharmacopeia of mineral waters adapted to cure the diseases incident to the southern climate and constitution. Thus, southerners came to imagine their physical environment paradoxically as the source of both healing and harming, as both the site of infection and the location of the cure.

Because of this paradoxical relationship, southerners did not view 'the environment' uniformly: they viewed particular elements as potentially useful or harmful depending on a constellation of factors. This discrimination of vision in turn meant that southerners looked to the waters themselves for direction in their therapeutic uses. In order to gainsay such usage, proprietors of the springs and other interested parties hired skilled scientists from southern universities to analyze the chemical and mineral content of the waters and to precisely measure their temperatures. Southern doctors would then 'decipher' this information for the lay public, articulating reasons and directions for the use of one spring or another for a particular illness. Of course, many of these explanations contradicted one another, and still others were motivated by reasons other than the humanitarian or scientific – but at the southern watering places, the waters, more than any philosophy or social reform movement, directed the cure.

In the Virginia springs region, the diversity of such specifically therapeutic waters gave southern hydropaths a vast catalogue of curative resources upon which to draw. Meanwhile, the prevailing belief among southern allopathic physicians that disease was rooted in the physical environment led them to argue that place-based disease could be removed by altering an environmental element, such as water or air. Thus, as southern hydropaths observed the springs' varying mineral contents, gas concentrations, and temperatures – not to mention their slightly different micro-climates, elevations, and air – they claimed for individual springs unique benefits (and sometimes drawbacks) in treating diseases associated with particular environmental qualities. Because each spring offered a unique composition of minerals, temperatures, and gaseousness, diseased bodies requiring more or less hydropathic stimulation could travel to the spring best suited to their particular situation; patients could also move from spring to spring, if necessary, as their conditions alleviated or as their constitutions became more or less 'excited' throughout the season. Physicians and other springs experts capitalized on this curative specificity by reminding their clientele that the variety of waters in the Virginia springs region – combined with the salubrious climate of the mountainous resorts – presented a panoply of remedies ideally suited to their particular complaints: 'when the agency of the greatest variety of Mineral Springs in the world may be obtained in connexion with climate,' Burke argued in 1842, 'our southern friends have inducements to visit us, which are not presented by any other region of the Union' (Burke 1842, 254). In these ways, southern medical experts and laypeople alike began to conceive of the springs region as a bountiful, diverse pharmacopeic resource for the healing of southern bodies.

Accordingly, southern water-cure experts sought to position the waters within the materia medica of orthodox medicine. In pamphlets and book-length works about the Virginia springs, these physicians reflect in their language use their imagination of the waters-as-medicine: they noted that certain waters were 'contraindicated' in some diseases and not others; they categorized some as 'diuretic,' while others were 'emetic' or 'sedating'; and they talked of 'prescribing' the waters in order to effect positive health changes. Such arguments were not merely rhetorical; southern physicians and lay people had very real concerns about the degenerative effects of the South's relentlessly hot climate upon their bodies. Many believed their systems more permanently 'relaxed' than those of their northern counterparts, and thus, that regular 'stimulation' via mineral or thermal waters was required to excite the body into a more balanced state. For southern medical men, then, mineral waters did not constitute 'alternative medicine,' but rather were important, individualized tools in the fighting of disease, particularly those diseases targeting southern constitutions or originating in southern climates.

No problem remained more pervasive for southerners than liver diseases, and it is to these afflictions that the Virginia sulphur waters seemed particularly adapted. Typically 'southern' maladies, such as malaria and yellow fever, were believed to negatively impact the liver, and 'bilious' complaints – believed to result from hot climates or from exposure to disease-carrying miasms – pepper the correspondence and journals of countless nineteenth-century white southerners. Testimonials from patients and physicians alike concurred that the White Sulphur and Red Sulphur Springs in particular offered unparalleled opportunities for healing the liver diseases that commonly plagued southerners. Similarly, doctors and patients argued for the value of bathing in thermal waters in treating southern complaints. A promotional writer for the Hot Springs boasted in 1860, 'In no class of human maladies have these waters been more eminently successful than in those which prevail in the Southern and South-western States.'[7] Patients and doctors alike testified to the power of the Hot Springs to act upon liver ailments particular to southerners: springs-goer R.N. Fox claimed in September 1845 that his 'severe attack of Bilious Fever which confined me to bed near eight weeks' was relieved after three or four 'spout' baths at the Hot Springs. Just 24 hours later, 'a very large quantity of most unhealthy bile was discharged, and the following day I felt entirely freed from every symptom of disease.'[8] Cincinnati physician Daniel Drake recorded a similarly rapid recovery in 1838:

> Another [patient at the Hot Springs] had derangements of the abdominal functions, [...] of two or three years' standing; the consequence of cholera, bilious fever, and ague, in a southern climate. In a few hours after using the hot bath, he had a bilious dejection, which had not occurred before for eight months; in four days, [...] all his symptoms gave way. (Drake 1838, 568–9)

This case study convinced Drake and, alongside other such experiences, doctors like him, that the 'Hot Springs of Virginia [we]re really and rapidly curative' (Drake 1838, 570). With both sulphur and thermal waters lying in close proximity to one another, the Virginia springs region seemed to these doctors and their patients peculiarly adapted for the healing of white southern bodies.

'The angry questions of the day': secession and slavery at the Springs

As sectionalism took hold of a greater proportion of the nation's people in both the North and South, elite white southerners came to see the mineral springs as much more than a healthful natural resource: they also offered a physical location for white southerners from across the South to congregate and together defend southern identity, customs, and institutions. With similar histories, values, and ideas about the future of the newly defined 'South,' elite white southerners converging at the springs created a political microcosm of their region and collectively forged a unified regional-'national' identity. Of course, slavery remained foremost among those topics uniting them. At the southern watering places, the peculiar institution maintained a strong presence through architectural elements that reinforced the plantation ideal; through the bodies of enslaved people working to ensure the smooth operations of day-to-day activities; through the private conversations and letters exchanged between white southern visitors; and through the staging of political events at the resorts.

Dell Upton and John Michael Vlach have convincingly argued that physical landscapes have the capacity to act as extensions of ideological processes (Upton 1988, 357; Vlach 1991; 1993, xiv, 2, 8). The architectural and agricultural choices on southern properties conspired to reinforce not only the master's primacy but also the hierarchical structures of power distribution that characterized the plantation economy more broadly. On large plantations, Upton argues, this hierarchical representation manifested itself as 'sequences of social barriers: rows of trees, terraces, dependencies, the kitchen [...] [the] portico, doorway, grand stair hall, chambers for waiting, chambers for formal talking, chambers for formal dining. The whole was a carefully orchestrated exercise in the definition of status; every barrier successfully passed was a mark of preference' (1988, 357). The springs resorts replicated this system of physical-social barriers to a tee, from the entry spaces of their 'big houses' to the layouts of their grounds. Upon arriving at a particular watering place, travelers typically proceeded past trees, gates, fountains, and outbuildings before reaching the central hotel, whose location and relationship to the rest of the grounds created a resonant parallel with the plantation 'big house' in the minds of white slave owners. And some resorts maintained actual 'gate-keeping' operations as well: the exclusive White Sulphur, for example, hired the notoriously tyrannical Major Baylis Anderson to fill this duty, and Anderson swiftly came to be known throughout elite white southern culture as the 'Metternich of the Mountains' for his totalitarian method of accepting or rejecting entire traveling parties seemingly at a whim. These physical and social 'checkpoints' mirrored the hierarchical structures southerners enacted and experienced in their home places.

During their stays at the springs, most white southerners resided in 'cabins' that were sprinkled throughout the property, sometimes laid out on orderly rows or 'streets.' These 'cabins' were not small, rustic houses, but rather very large and well-constructed brick homes of six or more rooms. The assignment of these accommodations also reflected the hierarchical organization of white southern society, as a traveling party would expect to receive a cabin on par with its social standing. Thus, the wealthiest white southerners would enjoy the larger and better-situated cabins, while those with fewer resources might share a cabin with another family. Because the central hotel was generally situated at the heart of the resort, some might argue that these cabins could have easily been interpreted as plantation 'outbuildings' or even as slave quarters. But the sturdy, permanent, and relatively large nature of these residences renders this interpretive possibility unlikely. Instead, the hierarchical assignment of cabin locations relied upon the external measures that were familiar to white southerners in their home towns and cities: those with the most wealth (often equated with those holding the largest numbers of slaves) or best connections received the best treatment.

However, proprietors of springs resorts went beyond these resonant and largely symbolic architectural reinforcements of the plantation ideal. In their catering to southern tastes, resort owners took care to give names to the cabins, other buildings, and 'streets' of the property that would appeal to white southerners' regional loyalties. At the White Sulphur Springs, for example, proprietor James Calwell named rows for Alabama, Louisiana, Baltimore, Carolina, Georgia, and Virginia. Meanwhile, at the Salt Sulphur, a 'Nullification Row' (Nicklin 1837, 208) paid homage to South Carolinian guests and to white southerners' burgeoning sense of states rights that the Nullification Crisis represented.[9] Such names suggest the geographical distribution of visitors to the springs: although genteel white southerners would almost certainly not turn 'Yankee' guests away from the Virginia watering places, these resorts likely did not receive many northern patrons.

Of course, the most obvious way in which the springs resorts resembled southern plantation systems was in the presence of enslaved people and free black servants. Promotional literature on the Virginia springs included inducements for white slave owners to bring their 'servants'[10] with them, offering reduced (often half-price) board and lodging for enslaved people. Proprietors most likely offered these reduced fees for enslaved people because they assumed that they would not 'take the waters,' that the reason for their presence was to provide service to their owners and not to receive treatment for disease. Moreover, the reduced fees acknowledged the subsequent reduction in labor that the resort owners themselves would otherwise have had to provide, although this aspect of the policy was never stated outright. If every slave-owning visitor brought a 'servant,' then the resort did not have to offer certain services, such as bringing water to private cabins, 'rubbing' and dressing patients after bathing, and providing equine and stage coach services. And because of the seasonal nature of work at the resorts, springs proprietors often faced labor shortages, so that guests bringing their own help proved desirable (Chambers 2002, 25). At the more fashionable resorts, such as the White Sulphur Springs, those white

14

southerners who brought along enslaved people were more likely to receive better service: Isaac Gorham Peck wrote in 1833 that people traveling in private coaches with 'servants' more frequently received the approving nod from that resort's formidable gatekeeper, thereby gaining admission to the resort when its accommodations were at capacity; George Featherstonhaugh corroborated this statement in 1844 (Featherstonhaugh 1844, 50). Once there, enslaved and free black servants at the springs provided music for the nightly dances, brought jugs of water to private cabins, and waited upon white guests at meal times, among countless other activities. While the precise number of enslaved and free black people present at the springs resorts – both those employed by the proprietors and those accompanying white travelers – remains unknown, if only half or even a third of a resort's visitors brought their 'servants,' the number must have been very large indeed.

Yet the presence of enslaved people is elided from virtually all visual and print culture of the period, and remarked upon only tangentially in letters and diaries. For example, one account records that the Salt Sulphur Springs opened in 1823 with slave quarters neighboring the two-story 'big house' (Brewster 1947, 97–8), although no visual or archival descriptions of these quarters (to the author's knowledge) exists. The surviving architectural plans of Virginia springs resorts do not depict slave quarters or separate springs for enslaved people, but brief remarks in the primary literature indicate that both sorts of facilities existed, at least at some of the larger and more popular sites. For example, the 1847 map of the White Sulphur reprinted in Moorman's *Virginia springs* includes the blacksmith, ballroom, neighboring tavern, ten pin alley, bathing houses, and stables, but it does not indicate the spring that enslaved people used here. In a throwaway comment easily missed amid a paragraph about a new species of snail discovered at the White Sulphur Spring, author Philip Nicklin ironically dubs this segregated spring the 'Black Sulphur,' and notes its comparatively humble springhouse:

> About twenty yards from the principal White Sulphur Spring is another of similar water under a plain shed, which a witty friend and fellow-townsman was wont to call the Black Sulphur Spring, because it was exclusively used by the Melanthropes. (Nicklin 1837, 179–80)

George Featherstonhaugh described this same segregated spring in 1844 in a similarly truncated manner:

> A few paces from [the main spring] is another reservoir of the water, surrounded with a curb-stone, where the negro servants assemble and drink in imitation of their masters, and out of which water is dipped for the use of the horses in the contiguous stables. (Featherstonhaugh 1844, 55)

Although this spring apparently existed in close proximity to the main spring at the White Sulphur, it appears on none of the maps and plans located for this study. Such scant comments demonstrate that enslaved people at the springs participated in the culture of taking the waters alongside white visitors – even though they were relegated to drinking water reserved for animals. And because white sojourners generally moved from one springs resort to another throughout the season, it is likely that enslaved people were present at many more resorts than the White Sulphur.

The question remains whether those enslaved people at the springs drank the waters because of their own ill health, because they wished to prevent disease, or for other reasons. The medical logic governing white southerners' use of the mineral springs rested on the concept of stimulating a body made languid by a hot climate, but that same logic understood black bodies as already ideally suited to hot climates, and thus, in no need of therapeutic stimulation. Because they were not 'native' to the South, white southerners argued, black bodies did not contract the same place-based diseases that white bodies did, and thus, could not be healed by those mineral waters peculiarly adapted to treat climatic and place-based diseases. Yet archival evidence reveals that at least some enslaved and free black people at the springs did use the waters for various ailments, at times exchanging labor for hydropathic treatment. In a letter dated 16. September 1831, Susannah Harrison Blain told her father that her party 'found Anthony on our return [to the White Sulphur] doing remarkably well, he says this water has worked miracles for him, that it works him <u>same as physick</u>: he finds employment in the neighbouring fields every day.' And at the Rockbridge Alum Springs, exchanging labor for treatment was an accepted – even a solicited – practice: the management there advertised that it would take in enslaved people suffering from scrofula and other skin diseases, granting them full access to the waters in exchange for their labor at the resort (Fishwick 1978, 212). Jerome Bonaparte, Jr.'s coachman convalesced for more than five weeks at the White Sulphur while his party waited for his recovery there; when they eventually left for the Warm Springs, the man required another fortnight before he fully recovered, which Bonaparte lamented: '[D]uring the whole time [. . .] he had been of no use at all to us,' he recorded in 1846 (Hoyt 1946, 129).

Such complaints about the 'usefulness' of enslaved and free black people often provided the occasion for white southerners at the springs to mention their presence – or as the case might be, their absence. In the dining room, springs visitors and proprietors frequently complained that the waiters did not work unless guests paid them bribes. William Burke noted that even though the kitchen at the White Sulphur seemed adequately supplied, visitors had trouble receiving full meals because of the prevalence of such bribery: 'As soon as the dishes are placed on the table, the private servants and those of the establishment that are bribed, seize upon the best of the eatables and place them as *private* property before their employers. It is a shameful abuse, and [. . .] the greatest evil at the White Sulphur' (Burke 1842, 102–3, emphasis in original). At other springs, there seemed to be a dearth of help when large crowds stuffed the resorts to capacity, and visitors reported that the servants were notoriously poor in quality and scant in quantity (Brewster 1947, 91). Any black person at the resort not seen as exercising a 'useful' purpose was liable to be enjoined to help white valetudinarians there, regardless of age or infirmity. Burke even argued that young black children at the Red Sweet could work as extra 'rubbers,' those who toweled off health-seekers after plunge baths: 'Where there are so many young negroes doing nothing,' he claimed, 'it would be no additional expense, and would greatly benefit invalid bathers' (Burke 1846, 116).

White visitors also used their complaints about poor service at the springs to uphold racist beliefs about the suitability of black people for enslavement. According to proslavery medical-social logic, free black servants presented a societal nuisance if not an outright danger to white people, while enslavement represented black people's 'proper' place. Some white visitors to the springs thus maintained that the poor service resulted from the status of resort-employed servants, who were typically free rather than enslaved. Even enslaved people under the care of more 'relaxed' owners could create behavioral problems that some proslavery physicians[11] denoted medical, or that ideologues denoted 'natural.' Susannah Harrison Blain reflected this logic when she wrote to her mother from the White Sulphur Springs that she 'recognized John White among the waiters,' who is 'an excellent servant under his present master *who is very strict*' (Blain, 24 August 1831, emphasis added), implying that he would not be so 'excellent' under a more lenient master. Reports of problems from free black servants at southern springs emphasized that their liberated status created those problems: 'there seems to be altogether free servants with a few exceptions,' Mary Brown wrote her husband from Buffalo Springs,

> and of course much wrongdoing among them[.] Mr Raine told me tonight he had the worst set he ever saw, but could not send them off – [...] told me that the servants in the dry room had broken [...] 35 dollars worth of crockery – + to-day 5 or 6 – a large salver + c – + he could not find out who did it –.[12]

Brown calls attention to the dual nature of the (perceived) 'problem' of the presence of free black people: their status naturally led to 'much wrongdoing,' and yet the scarcity of workers meant that proprietors 'could not send them off.' Among a certain set of white slave owners, this attitude toward free black workers was so pervasive that despite shortages of labor (and the resultant encouragement from proprietors, via financial incentives, to bring enslaved servants to the springs), they expressed reluctance to bring those servants with them. Fearing that free black influence would 'corrupt' and spoil enslaved people – that after their time at the springs slaves might not be content with farm work – some cautious white slave owners opted to travel without their enslaved attendants (Lewis 2001, 41–3).

Just as they shared notes on the perceived 'dangerousness' of free black servants, groups of white slave owners congregating at the Virginia springs from different southern localities used the space of the springs to consolidate proslavery ideologies. The rural, mountainous resorts remained geographically isolated from most urban political activities, but special public events and visits from political celebrities such as Henry Clay engaged springs-goers in the issues of the day, just as private correspondence included references to current news and politics. Although a letter writer to the *Richmond Examiner* recorded in 1848 that 'by general consent the angry questions of the day [were] avoided'[13] – that social life at the springs steered clear of sensitive topics in favor of light-hearted gossip and flirting – springs-goers apparently (and eagerly) discussed several 'angry questions' throughout the nineteenth century. John Skinner's 1847 diary contains numerous references to the ongoing Mexican War, recording that 'The Southern men with whom I have conversed are dead against the Wilmot Proviso,[14] and equally dead against the acquisition of any more territory' (Bishko 1972, 181). Susannah Harrison Blain wrote her mother from the White Sulphur Springs just seven days after the conclusion of Nat Turner's rebellion, 'Are you not rendered uneasy by the affair in South Hampton? some persons here are a good deal excited' (Blain 30 August 1831). In August 1835, prominent Whigs in Virginia held a public dinner at the Buffalo Lithia Springs to honor two party leaders from North Carolina and Virginia (Keanan et al. 1835). Ardent secessionist Edmund Ruffin wrote in 1856 that he 'used every suitable occasion to express my opinion, & the grounds thereof, that the slave-holding states should speedily separate from the others, & form a separate confederacy' (quoted in Chambers 2002, 176). Indeed, Ruffin found the Virginia springs 'the proper salon for all he had to say,' and did not refrain from discussing disunion with anyone at the springs who might listen, including the governor of South Carolina, when the two men were both guests at the

White Sulphur Springs in August 1859 (Fishwick 1978, 35). And in John Pendleton Kennedy's *Swallow barn*, one of the more popular works of antebellum southern fiction, the travels to the springs of protagonist Frank Meriwether are solely motivated by the desire to share his opinions with the other guests congregated at the resorts: noting that he travels – somewhat reluctantly – to the springs 'every autumn,' the narrator explains that the 'upper country is not much to his taste, and would not be endured by him if it were not for [...] the opportunity this concourse [of people] affords him for discussion of opinions' (Kennedy 1832, 34). Far from anomalous, these examples instead illustrate the active engagement of springs-goers in the current events and 'angry questions' of their day.

Such engagement only continued through the late 1840s – particularly during the election of 1848 – and throughout the 1850s. Virginia Whigs arranged for a political debate to be held at Buffalo Springs in August 1848, inviting 'the opposite party to a discussion of the political issues of the day' (Tazewell et al. 1848); they did so with a view of promoting the Whig presidential ticket of Zachary Taylor and Millard Fillmore. Held at the height of the springs season in late August, this political debate demonstrates the use of the springs venue, with its large numbers of guests, as a forum for the promotion of those political ideas favored by white southerners. Also in August 1848, the Fauquier White Sulphur Springs hosted a Democratic 'mass meeting,' where a number of proslavery southerners gave speeches encouraging Virginians to preserve southern interests by voting for the Democratic ticket; these speakers feared that Taylor, the Whig candidate, could not win, and that southerners' support for him would inadvertently lead to the election of Free Soil candidate Martin Van Buren.[15] The springs provided an ideal venue for these large political meetings, as the presence of hundreds of guests – most of them proslavery – ensured an extensive and receptive audience to Democratic and Whig principles. Thus, the Virginia springs provided not an escape from the 'angry questions of the day' but rather a place that mitigated that 'anger' through the relative homogeneity of the guests' political views. With the numbers of northern visitors declining throughout the period, political activists could expect an audience at the springs composed primarily of fellow slave-owning southerners.

Through cultural apparatuses such as reduced fees for enslaved people and attention to hierarchical social systems, through cultural constructs such as the perceived 'dangerousness' of free black servants, and through cultural performances such as political events, slave-owning southerners created a space at the springs where their medical, social, and natural philosophies came together to justify continued enslavement and to bolster support for the distinctiveness of the collective southern body, which was gradually evolving into a body politic. At the same time, the proliferation of the idea that the waters were 'peculiarly adapted' to the treatment of particularly 'southern' diseases, alongside the promotion of a racial logic that asserted the usefulness of warm southern waters for diseased white bodies, enabled white southerners to claim individual bodily distinctiveness by matching climate, disease, and cure in one broad region: while the southern environment might cause diseases, a beneficent southern nature would also provide the means to cure them. As slave-owning southerners traveled to the Virginia waters, mountains, and salubrious climate at the heart of this closed system, they recreated the physical and intellectual structures necessary for justifying slavery and for imagining an independent, 'wholesome,' and healthful southern nation.

Acknowledgements

The author would like to gratefully acknowledge the following libraries and institutions for granting access to their outstanding collections and for providing financial support: the Southern Historical Collection and the Rare Book Collection of Wilson Library, University of North Carolina, Chapel Hill; the Virginia Historical Society in Richmond, Virginia; the Rackham Graduate School and the University of Michigan, Ann Arbor; the Andrew Mellon Foundation; and the William Reese Company. She would also like to thank Susan Scott Parrish and Alexandra Minna Stern for their helpful feedback on earlier versions of the manuscript, and Cristiana Bastos and Harish Naraindas for their gracious support of this project.

Statement on ethics: Because the subjects of this research paper are historical figures, no ethical conflicts exist. All archival sources are used with permission of the holding institutions.

Conflict of interest: none.

Notes

1. Burke's use of the adjective 'ruddy' to describe the healthfulness of blood also implies an imagined white audience, since 'ruddy' typically referred to a 'fresh' or 'healthy' 'redness of complexion' (*Oxford English Dictionary*). Thus, the 'children' of Virginia – the 'native' Americans – are implicitly and exclusively coded as white, not as American Indians or enslaved black people.
2. Berkeley Springs at various points in its history was also known as 'Warm Springs,' 'Frederick Springs,' and 'Bath.'
3. Which landscapes counted as 'sickly' and which as 'healthy' oscillated throughout the eighteenth century. For example, in the early 1700s, many white southerners viewed the coastal city of Charleston as a safe haven, but by the 1790s, they had come to view it as dangerously pestilential. By the end of the century, urban – especially low-lying urban – places were firmly situated in the category of the 'sickly,' while cooler, mountainous places were deemed 'salubrious.' For more on the healthfulness of particular landforms, see Valencius (2002).
4. Lewis (2001), Chambers (2002), Fishwick (1978), Gill (2002), and Shepard (1987).
5. Resorts in Arkansas, Georgia, Kentucky, Missouri, North Carolina, Tennessee, and Texas added to that number, though none of these would come to equal the fame and perceived curative value of the Virginia springs. For more on these springs, see Bullard (2004), Tichi (2001), and Valenza (2000).
6. This sentence also echoes the arguments of Joan Burbick (1994), who in *Healing the republic* claims that the health of the early republic could be indexed by the health of its citizenry.
7. From *Some account of the medicinal properties [...]* (1860, 9).
8. From *Some account of the medicinal properties [...]* (1860, 30–1).
9. The Nullification Crisis of 1832–33, when the state of South Carolina 'nullified' federal tariff legislation, created a standoff between the state and the federal government; this 'states-rights' protest eventually led to the formation of the Whig party, which remained popular with white southerners, particularly with the former 'nullifiers' and those opposing what they saw as an autocratic president in Andrew Jackson.
10. The word 'servant' was almost always used as a euphemism for 'slave' by elite white slave owners and by those who catered to them, such as springs proprietors.
11. One such physician includes Samuel Cartwright, who argued tirelessly in medical journals for a biological basis to race, and consequently, for a biological justification of black inferiority. See Cartwright (1846–47) and (1851) for examples of this line of argumentation.
12. Brown, n.d. [pre-1861].
13. Stokes (1848).
14. The Wilmot Proviso, which passed the House in 1846 but did not succeed in the Senate (where southern votes had more influence), would have banned slavery in

any territory annexed from Mexico as a result of the (then-ongoing) Mexican-American War.

15. See *The Daily Union* (1848). Van Buren's candidacy and possible win was such a lightning rod to proslavery southerners that author Nathaniel Beverley Tucker imagined his continued presidency as triggering the secession of southern states. In *The partisan leader* (1836), penned after Van Buren's election as the eighth President of the United States, Tucker foresees a fictional world of 1856, where Van Buren is serving out his fourth term as an antislavery president. In a prescient imaginative move, Tucker has the slave-holding states secede immediately after Van Buren is elected President, foreshadowing the actions of the same states just 24 years later upon Abraham Lincoln's election. The author would like to thank John Miller for bringing this novel to her attention.

16. Abbreviations in the list of references correspond to the following: RB-UNC: Rare Book Collection, Wilson Library, University of North Carolina, Chapel Hill. VHS: Virginia Historical Society, Richmond, Virginia.

References[16]

'Account of George Washington with Martha Parke Custis.' 12 September 1769. George Bolling Lee Papers, 1707–1790, Section 2. Mss1 L5114 a19, VHS.

Bishko, Lucretia Ramsey, ed. 1972. John S. Skinner visits the Virginia springs, 1847. *Virginia Magazine of History and Biography* 80 (April): 158–92.

Blain, Susannah Isham Harrison. 24 August 1831. Letter to Mary (Randolph) Harrison [mother]. White Sulphur [Springs]. Harrison Family Papers, 1725–1907, Section 8. Mss1 H2485 c669, VHS.

Blain, Susannah Isham Harrison. 30 August 1831. Letter to Mary (Randolph) Harrison [mother]. White Sulphur [Springs]. Harrison Family Papers, 1725–1907, Section 8. Mss1 H2485 c670, VHS.

Blain, Susannah Isham Harrison. 16 September 1831. Letter to Randolph Harrison [father]. White Sulphur [Springs]. Harrison Family Papers, 1725–1907, Section 1. Mss1 H2485 c2, VHS.

Brewster, Lawrence Fay. 1947. Summer migrations and resorts of South Carolina low-country planters. In *Historical papers of the Trinity College Historical Society*, Series XXVI, 3–134. Durham: Duke University Press.

Bridenbaugh, Carl. 1946. Baths and watering places of colonial America. *William and Mary Quarterly* (Third Series) 3.2 (April): 151–81.

Brown, Mary Virginia Early. n.d. [pre-1861]. Letter to James L. Brown [husband]. Buffalo [Lithia] Springs. Early Family Papers, 1798–1903, Section 10, Folder 3. Mss1 Ea765 a128, VHS.

Bullard, Loring. 2004. *Healing waters: Missouri's historic mineral springs and spas*. Columbia, MO: University of Missouri Press.

Burbick, Joan. 1994. *Healing the republic: The language of health and the culture of nationalism in nineteenth-century America*. Cambridge studies in American literature and culture 82. Ed. Eric Sundquist. Cambridge: Cambridge University Press.

Burke, William. 1842. *The mineral springs of western Virginia: With remarks on their use, and the diseases to which they are applicable*. New York: Wiley and Putnam.

Burke, William. 1846. *The mineral springs of western Virginia: With remarks on their use, and the diseases to which they are applicable. [...]. by William Burke. 2nd ed., revised, corrected, and enlarged*. New York: Wiley and Putnam.

Burke, William. 1851. *The mineral springs of Virginia; With remarks on their use, the diseases to which they are applicable, and in which they are contra-indicated. [...]. by William Burke*. Richmond, VA: Morris & brother.

Cartwright, Samuel A. 1846–47. Cartwright on southern medicine. *New Orleans Medical and Surgical Journal* III: 259–72.

Cartwright, Samuel A. 1851. The diseases and physical peculiarities of the negro race. In *Southern Medical Reports* Vol. II. Ed. Erasmus Darwin Fenner, M.D., 421–29. New Orleans and New York: S. Samuel and William Wood.

Cayleff, Susan E. 1988. Gender, ideology, and the water-cure movement. In *Other healers: Unorthodox medicine in America*. Ed. Norman Gevitz, 82–98. Baltimore: Johns Hopkins University Press.

Chambers, Thomas A. 2002. *Drinking the waters: Creating an American leisure class at nineteenth-century mineral springs*. Washington, DC: Smithsonian Institution Press.

The Daily Union. 1848. Democratic mass meeting at Fauquier. August 23.

Drake, Daniel. 1838. Mineral springs of Virginia: Notices of the Blue Sulphur, and Hot Springs, of the state of Virginia. Article VIII. *The Western Journal of the Medical and Physical Sciences*, Edited and published, quarterly, by the medical faculty of the Cincinnati College 11, no. 44 (January, February, and March): 565–70.

Featherstonhaugh, George W. 1844. *Excursion through the slave states, from Washington on the Potomac to the frontier of Mexico; with sketches of popular manners and geological notices*. London: John Murray.

Fishwick, Marshall William. 1978. *Springlore in Virginia*. Bowling Green: Popular Press, Bowling Green State University.

Gill, Harold B. 2002. Taking the cure. *Colonial Williamsburg: The Journal of the Colonial Williamsburg Foundation* 24, no. 2 (Summer): 74–80.

Green, Harvey. 1986. *Fit for America: Health, fitness, sport and American society*. New York: Pantheon Books.

Hoyt, William D., Jr., ed. 1946. Journey to the springs, 1846. [Jerome Bonaparte, Jr.] *Virginia magazine of history and biography* 54 (April): 119–36.

Jefferson, Thomas. 1785, 1787. *Notes on the state of Virginia*. Ed. Frank Shuffelton. New York: Penguin, 1999.

Keanan, Erasmus; Benjamin Sims; Thomas M. Nelson; et al. ['Committee.'] 15 July 1835. Letter to William F. Gordon, Esq. Mecklenburg C[ourt]H[ouse], Virginia. Armistead Churchill Gordon Papers, 1705–1957, Section 1. Mss1 G6532 b2, VHS.

Kennedy, John Pendleton. 1832. *Swallow barn; or, a sojourn in the Old Dominion*, ed. Lucinda H. MacKethan. The Library of Southern Civilization Series, ed. Lewis P. Simpson. Baton Rouge: Louisiana State University Press, 1986.

Lewis, Charlene M. Boyer. 2001. *Ladies and gentlemen on display: Planter society at the Virginia springs, 1790–1860*. Charlottesville: University Press of Virginia.

Moorman, J[ohn]. J[ennings]. 1847. *The Virginia springs: With their analysis and some remarks on their character, together with a directory for the use of the White Sulphur water, and an account of the diseases to which it is applicable; to which is added, a review of a portion of Wm. Burke's book on the mineral springs of western Virginia, etc. by John J. Moorman*. Philadelphia: Lindsay & Blakiston. VHS.

Nicklin, Philip Houlbrooke. [pseud. Peregrine Prolix.] 1837. *Letters descriptive of the Virginia springs: The roads leading thereto, and the doings thereat. Collected, corrected, annotated, and edited by Peregrine Prolix. With a map of Virginia*, 2nd edn. Philadelphia: H.S. Tanner. VHS.

Peck, Isaac Gorham. 19 July – 16 August 1833. Diary. [Typed transcription.] Isaac Gorham Peck Papers, 1822–1838, Section 1. Mss1 P3354 b1, VHS.

Shalinsky, Audrey C. 1985. Thermal springs as folk curing mechanisms. *Folklore Forum* 18: 32–58.

[Shepard, E. Lee.] 1987. Introd. to *First resorts: A visit to Virginia's springs. An exhibition*. Richmond: Virginia Historical Society.

Some account of the medicinal properties of the Hot Springs, Virginia; also an analysis of the water, with cases of cure of gout, rheumatism, diseases of the liver, paralysis, neuralgia, chronic diarroea, enlarged glands, old in[j]uries, deafness, etc., etc. 1860. Richmond, VA. Printed by Chas. H. Wynne. Southern Pamphlet #2614, RB-UNC.

Stokes, Jacob. 1848. Fauquier White Sulphur Springs. Letter to the *Richmond Examiner*. August 27.

Tazewell, Littleton; A.C. Morton; G.A. Wilson; et al. [Committee.] August 1848. Letter to Hon. William B. Preston, Clarksville [Virginia]. Preston Family Papers, 1773–1862, Section 14. Mss1 P9267 d474, VHS.

Tichi, Cecilia. 2001. *Embodiment of a nation: Human form in American places*. Cambridge, MA: Harvard University Press.

Tucker, Nathaniel Beverley. 1836. *The partisan leader*. Ed. Carl Bridenbaugh. New York: Knopf, 1933.

Upton, Dell. 1988. White and black landscapes in eighteenth-century Virginia. In *Material life in America, 1600–1860*, Ed. Robert Blair St. George, 357–69. Boston: Northeastern University Press.

Valencius, Conevery. 2002. *The health of the country: How American settlers understood themselves and their land*. New York: Basic Books.

Valenza, Janet Mace. 2000. *Taking the waters in Texas: Springs, spas, and fountains of youth*. Austin: University of Texas Press.

Vlach, John Michael. 1991. Plantation landscapes of the antebellum South. In *Before freedom came: African-American life in the antebellum South*, ed. D.C. Campbell, Jr. and Kym S. Rice, 21–49. Richmond and Charlottesville: The Museum of the Confederacy and University Press of Virginia.

Vlach, John Michael. 1993. *Back of the big house: The architecture of plantation slavery*. The Fred W. Morrison series in southern studies. Chapel Hill: University of North Carolina Press.

Seeking 'energy' vs. pain relief in spas in Brazil (Caldas da Imperatriz) and Portugal (Termas da Sulfúrea)

Maria Manuel Quintela

Department of Community Health, Nursing School of Lisbon (ESEL), Portugal; CRIA/ISCTE-IUL, Lisbon, Portugal

This paper is a comparative ethnography of the therapeutic practices at two different spa locations: Caldas da Imperatriz, SC, Brazil, and Termas da Sulfúrea in Cabeço de Vide, Portugal. The comparison reveals the existence of contrasting 'explanatory models' held by the spa-goers as well as by the official medical systems. In the Portuguese context this model is highly medicalized; in the Brazilian case, spa treatments are viewed as 'alternative' or 'complementary' therapy and are also related to religious philosophies. Each model corresponds to a different idiom expressing certain experiences and world views, one focusing on 'pains' (*dores*) and the other on 'energy' (*energia*), the former leading to the rationale of 'curing', the latter to the notion of 'energizing'. In this paper the author intends to analyze and contrast the categories found in these models, which originate from different conceptions of health, illness and healing for Brazilian and Portuguese spa-goers.

Introduction

In Portugal, as in some other European countries, the therapeutic use of hot springs is recognized as a specialization of biomedicine called 'medical hydrology' and its activities are known as *thermalism* or 'water cures'.[1] In Brazil, however, it is considered an 'alternative' or 'complementary' practice to medicine. Based on ethnographic research conducted in Portuguese and Brazilian hot water spas, the author intends to compare and analyze the central categories of 'pains' and 'energy' in explanatory models of thermal treatment by spa therapy consumers which, in turn, refer to different conceptions of health, illness and treatment.

The spas[2] or *termas* bring together very different realities: 'belief' and 'science'; 'popular medicine' and biomedicine; the chemical/medicinal or 'miraculous' properties attributed to the waters; asceticism and sociability; suffering and enjoyment; as well as the aspects of healing and leisure themselves. An analysis of thermal practices cannot ignore the recreational and therapeutic aspects that are inherent in thermalism. The intersection and juxtaposition of all these aspects makes the study of spas a stimulating project.

The comparative analysis of spa practices in two geographic and cultural contexts also enables us to overcome the opposition between 'medicines' (bio-medicine and ethno-medicine, including the so-called 'folk' or 'traditional') and the 'therapies' (scientific, alternative, complementary). While this opposition has circulated since the inception of studies in medical anthropology or the anthropology of health or illness, the conceptions of treatment and healing cut across it. In addition, the transformation of medical paradigms has historically determined the relationship between hot mineral water usage and health. It is therefore impossible to separate the study of thermal practices and thermalism from the history of medicine and therapy as Georges Weisz (1995, 2001) and Roy Porter (1990) have demonstrated.

The data presented here derive from ethnographic research conducted as part of PhD dissertation work (Quintela 2008). Fieldwork in Brazil was carried out over 12 months between 2002 and 2003, and focused on Caldas da Imperatriz, a spa setting situated in the state of Santa Catarina in southern Brazil. In Portugal, research was carried out in Termas da Sulfúrea (Cabeço de Vide), located in the south of Portugal, from September to November 2003, and also included visits to other Portuguese spas as part of PhD dissertation work.[3] Previous studies in Termas de São Pedro do Sul (Quintela 1999, 2001) also contributed to understanding how Portuguese thermalism and its practices were shaped, which are relevant to the argument of this paper.[4] In addition, Portuguese thermalism was changing quickly and Termas da Sulfúrea was in the process of making a transition towards newer Portuguese spa trends (Quintela 2008). It had the appearance of a 'classic thermalism' spa with older buildings and equipment, but at the same time had begun building a new bath house, that was inaugurated in May 2007.[5] In Brazil, Caldas da Imperatriz was chosen for being somehow equivalent to Termas de São Pedro do Sul in Portugal: it was associated with the beginnings of thermalism in the country and offered a point of reference for understanding the shaping of thermalism in Brazil. Another reason for choosing this setting relates to the fact that it dates back to the period when Brazil was a Portuguese colony (1818), bringing some elements regarding the circulation of knowledge during the colonial period to this study.

Comparison of therapeutic spa practices revealed two contexts with differences that were relevant on various levels: in Portugal, thermalism was included in the official health system as a medical specialization (biomedicine); in Brazil it was not included in the official Unified System of Health (SUS) and was classified as a practice associated with alternative or complementary medicine. Development of the thermalism process in both countries originated from the different historical traditions of mineral water use (Quintela 2004). In this paper the author will examine the medicalization[6] of thermalism and analyze thermal experiences in the two contexts starting from the triad of thermalism-medicine-tourism.

The thermalism-medicine-tourism triad

Some medical literature dating from late nineteenth-century Brazil and Portugal reveals the importance given to chemical analysis of mineral waters, their 'scientific' treatment, and of registering the clinical data of patients who used them. This made it possible to establish a relationship between the waters' chemical and physical properties and its therapeutic effects. This medical practice developed into a field of medical knowledge that began the process of its legitimization as a science in the second half of the nineteenth-century and what became the discipline of medical hydrology in the twentieth-century (Weisz 1995, 2001). Nevertheless, the development of medical hydrology in the two countries took different directions. In Portugal, the Institutes of Hydrology and Climatology were founded[7] with one of their purposes being to offer medical hydrology courses with the subject appearing in other medical curriculums; in Brazil, the subject was only taught at the medical schools of Rio de Janeiro and Minas Gerais and was then suppressed in the 1950s. This is one of the reasons why thermalism in Brazil is different from that in Portugal.

The discipline was responsible for medicalizing thermal settings and practices. In the Portuguese case, legislation itself did so via surveillance and sanitary control of bathing establishments and their entire surroundings, including lodging – hotels and guest houses – with the aim of promoting 'hygiene' in the entire thermal area. It should be noted that Portuguese legislation regarding thermal activity (1919) gave the medical directors of thermal institutions responsibility for publicizing the respective region in order to promote tourism.

The case of Termas da Sulfúrea in Portugal illustrates these differences. Here, the medicalization process began in late nineteenth-century with the construction of a thermal bath house whose access was subject to medical control. This increased throughout the twentieth-century with the appearance of doctors-in-residence specialized in medical hydrology. In the Brazilian case of Caldas da Imperatriz, the author witnessed an inverse process with the thermal hospital – in operation since 1884 – being transformed into a hotel. This hospital belonged to the province of Santa Catarina, and at the end of the nineteenth-century the provincial governor himself mentioned in his reports the need to associate the hospital with other dimensions besides curative ones, giving the example of starting a restaurant. Economic motives were also the reason for reformulating the building's function. A private company was awarded the concession to turn it into a thermal hotel not just for patients and without a doctor-in-residence. The hotel remains there today. The data suggest that the Caldas da Imperatriz setting developed during the twentieth-century at the margins of medicine and was geared more towards tourism development. According to the relationship established between the three dimensions of the triad thermalism-medicine-tourism and the weight of each, thermal locations were built, oscillating between medicine and tourism. The extent to which thermal practices are organized and experienced in a medicalized way reflects this.

Spas are places for leisure and healing (Mackaman 1998) where thermalism and tourism overlap. Depending on their level of organization, host populations receive guests – the spa-goers – in a set of infrastructures ranging from bath houses, to restaurants, to stores, to recreational facilities, as part of a relational phenomenon (Smith 1989). This reinforces the idea that medicine and tourism were associated in those thermal settings of greatest prominence in the twentieth-century, this relationship having fomented thermalism and development.

Spa practices: between healing and leisure

Ethnographic observation made it possible to identify thermal practices in these contexts today and to analyze how medicalization determines the organization and structure of the spa visit – the 'season' or 'fortnight' – and the thermal experiences of spa-goers (*termalistas*, *aquistas*, *hóspedes*) or guests.

In regards to the two contexts analyzed, the Portuguese spas showed evidence of medicalization, or even 'hospitalization,' while that was not evident in the Brazilian spa.

Two temporal vectors ritually organized the period of stay at the spa: 'treatment' time and 'leisure' time, which could take place at the same or at different establishments, depending on the concepts of 'treatment' and 'leisure' themselves. Whether these two activities were considered belonging to separate social spheres or an integrated practice reflected how thermal treatment was conceived and experienced and how space and time of thermal practices were organized in the two countries, whether joined or separated.

As the author mentioned above, thermal practices in Portugal take place in spaces similar to those of a hospital designated in these specific cases as bath houses (and in some cases visitors say 'I am going to the baths', 'I am going to the spa'). It is here that thermal and balneotherapeutic treatments take place throughout the duration of the spa stay. In the Portuguese case, this is usually a fortnight (15 days) or a minimum of 12 days (the number of days required for the health system to contribute to the cost of treatment). This varies according to social and economic reasons as well as the health sub-system to which the spa-goer belongs.

> This isn't vacation, I look at this like the hospital, we're being treated, right? We're being treated, at the hospital everybody stays in the ward, here [at the spa] everybody has their own room, and people get together with others. But I don't consider this a vacation. Going to France, like I did, going to Disneyland is vacation. It's not a sacrifice [coming to the spa], only monetarily, because it does me good. (R., age 54, widow, Sulfúrea)

The spa-goers at these spas are predominately women, as indicated in the clinical reports and corresponding to national statistics on spa visits. They belong to an over-40 age group and are on average between 65 and 74 years old. Some of these women come to the spas alone regardless of their marital status (married, widowed or single). The male spa-goers are usually married, visiting with their wives, most merely as chaperones, or sometimes undergoing treatment for 'sinusitis', 'bronchitis' or 'rhinitis'. The main reasons women give for seeking treatment is 'pains' and 'rheumatism'.

Visitors to Portuguese spas must go through a rite of passage from being guests to spa-goers. After visiting a doctor and describing their symptoms they are given a 'prescription' for water to be taken in the form of immersion, shower or vapor. Depending on the state of the spa-goer's health, the doctor prescribes a water temperature and treatment time (in minutes, with the average being about 15) as well as the number of treatments (in days).

The spa-goers refer to the set of thermal techniques employed during the fortnight as treatments or baths. In this establishment they offer various balneotherapy techniques: 'immersion bath'; '*Vidáqua*'; 'douche mouve'; 'Bertholaix' and 'inhalotherapy' etc.[8] There are diverse forms of using and consuming mineral water: immersion, ingestion, vapor, inhalation and emanation. It is indicated that 'treatments' must be carried out in bathing attire (bathing cabinets) and with a bathing cap. All treatments involve balneotherapy assistants who control the water temperature and length of treatment, and administer such balneotherapeutic techniques. After the baths, the spa-goers rest in reclining chairs in the 'resting room' or in the 'cooling room' for a minimum of 20 to 30 minutes. Some users spend up to an hour there and use the time to chat with their 'colleagues'.

In the waiting room, the author observed bath clothing (robes, slippers, bathing suits, track suits) and listened to the conversations between the spa-goers. These conversations combine talk of the 'need for care' and effectiveness of the 'treatments'. The primary concern is: 'don't catch a chill'.

> It is not enough to go there [to the spa], it is necessary to take special care not to catch cold, not catch a chill, to rest . . . Otherwise it would not be necessary to go to spas and undergo the treatment. (MF, age 78, Sulfúrea)

They also classify the waters as 'very good' and compare spas sites and mineral waters on a sensorial scale (heat, smell, taste) discussing their therapeutic properties, specialties and efficacy against skin, rheumatic and respiratory diseases, with some of them even recognizing that 'the waters don't heal, but relieve the pains!'

The bathers also discuss their treatments, diseases and the pains they suffer from, their doctors, the uses and efficacy of medicines. One of their justifications for having the 'fortnight' and for using mineral water as a 'natural medicine' is the inefficacy of chemical medicines: 'I take lots of medicines and they do nothing . . . ' The illness most often mentioned is 'rheumatism' (*reumatismo*), and the pains (*dores*) it causes. In some way it is revealing that, in the past as well as now, rheumatism (along with some skin and respiratory diseases) is still the main motive for undergoing thermal treatment, possibly suggesting the inability of biomedical knowledge to understand its causes and to offer a cure. The evolution of the relationship between 'thermal cure' and rheumatism can also be explored as a possible explanation for reconfigurations in Portuguese thermalism, depending on the value rheumatologists have given to this therapeutic practice either as 'medicine' or as 'placebo'.

At Portuguese spas, the spa-goers, predominately women, return to their lodgings after resting in the bath house and retire to their beds where they remain for the same period of time referred to above and for the same reason. The time spent on this ritual is one of the reasons given for scheduling treatment times and a source of tension among the staff. Treatment is scheduled according to availability. Nevertheless, the spa-goers usually ask to schedule treatment for the morning, the reason being that they want a 'free afternoon' to be able to 'go out'. Such situations cause the staff to express attitudes affirming the boundaries between the spaces for treatment and leisure: 'but did you come here to be treated or for a jaunt?', 'this place here is for treatment!' What does *tratar* (to treat) mean in this context?[9]

Tratar ('to treat') in these Portuguese spas is understood as the group of activities centered on the so-called 'treatments', 'baths', but which goes beyond the physical space of the bath house. This is because the ritual is only considered complete after resting is finished, continuing in the lodgings for a period of an hour. The spa-goers say they rest in bed, 'for all of the sweat to come out'. Nevertheless, after this they change clothes and a new 'jaunt' stage begins. A 'jaunt' ranges from taking a small walk, to taking a trip by car or bus, depending on available economic means.

The bath houses (*balneários*) are buildings independent from lodging and therefore their only purpose is 'treatments'. At the Termas de São Pedro do Sul there are plenty of tourism infrastructures (hotels, pools), organized recreational activities called 'spa entertainment' in public spaces at parks (dances, popular music concerts, movies) and tourism routes in the region. In the particular case of Termas da Sulfúrea, tourism (or its infrastructures) was practically non-existent up until the time fieldwork was carried out (2003). However, the local thermal landscape underwent changes at the time and tourist infrastructures (inn, hotel) appeared as well as a new bath building with updated thermal equipment, reinforcing the argument of the importance of the thermalism-medicine-tourism triad.

In Brazil, the 'baths' and the 'season' take place at the Hotel Caldas da Imperatriz. Length of stay varies widely according to guests' intentions. Stays at the thermal hotel vary from one week to one month. Weekend guests and those only staying for three or four days do so for leisure as part of other tourist activities in the region, including organized sports such as rafting and canoeing, or religious ones such as visiting Brother Hugolino[10] for a 'health blessing' or Mother Paulina. Pamphlets on regional tourism feature all of these products as well as Hotel Caldas da Imperatriz, the spa and the 'hot waters'. A 'season' refers to visits of no less than ten days, the period considered effective by those guests whose aim is 'health treatment'.

In this Brazilian thermal hotel – in contrast to the Portuguese spas studied – thermal activities, namely the baths, take place within the establishment. The admissions procedure is identical to that of any other hotel. The particularity of this one happens to be that it has thermal water baths. There is no doctor present and guests have free access to the baths. The number of baths taken is up to the criteria of each guest, according to their reasons and intentions for bathing. Baths are taken in marble bathtubs, in (six) individual cabinets.

The majority of the guests interviewed were women, with most aged 60–69, followed by those aged 70–79. Most guests had four to six years of education, followed by those with over 12 years. The majority of guests were from the southern Brazilian states of Paraná, Rio Grande do Sul and Santa Catarina.

Most guests interviewed alluded to 'the waters' (warm, natural, 'energizing') as the main reason for their stay, followed by 'the energy of the place', the hotel's 'family-like' hospitality where 'good food' and the 'natural' stand out, with their aim being 'energizing', 'resting', 'retiring', and 'taking care of health'. Baths can be taken according to the user's will and aims: therapeutic, relaxation and/or recreation, pure pleasure, well-being, 'energizing'. But depending on 'how the body reacts to the baths', guests decide how many baths to take, whether daily, or overall, so that they are effective. Most frequently two or three baths are taken daily: one before breakfast, one before afternoon tea (6–7 pm) and another before going to bed. Guests attribute the therapeutic efficacy to the water's properties: its 'warmness', 'natural' quality and 'energy'.

The option to stay in the thermal setting of Caldas da Imperatriz does not depend for the most part on medical advice. Nevertheless, guests often reiterate certain precautions and things to avoid when using the thermal baths or ingesting mineral water, repeating some of the language found in older medical literature about 'not catching a chill', the number of baths, rest and food. In the opinion of the guests, the thermal visit signifies bathing, rest, self-communion, daily exercise ('the walk'), restoring 'energy', visiting Brother Hugolino and 'getting away from it all'.

For guests, the 'season' is a set of interrelated recreational, religious and therapeutic activities not allocated to separate social spheres, in contrast with the Portuguese cases examined.

'Pains' (*dores*) and 'energy' (*energia*): explanatory models for thermal treatment

In the Brazilian and Portuguese thermal contexts the author encountered two contrasting attitudes supported on different references to health and illness – one based on the cult of health and a set of practices to care for the body (the eternal youth), to maintain it and 'to energize' it; the other based on illness, a routine experience of pain (Kleinman 1994) that must be eliminated or relieved. This is the basis for the expression 'treating one's health', and not illness, used in the Brazilian spa. The author might suggest that 'taking care of health' is, from a holistic perspective, also 'treating one's illness' whether eliminating or reducing the ailments it causes. These two forms of medicalization, one focusing on health and the other on illness, justify the different 'explanatory models' (Kleinman 1980) of thermal treatment.

The experience of the fortnight or season briefly described above reflects the higher or lower extent to which the spa location is medically organized, and the reasons spa-goers and guests give for seeking these types of places illustrate this. In the Portuguese spas studied, spa-goers seek 'relief from the pains' as illustrated in the narrative by Rosa, age 54:

> The waters are good, because they relieve my pains (*dores*). That's why they are good. After three weeks I notice improvement, I can already do things that used to hurt and I didn't do before, and I start to do them, the pains disappear, go, go away...

In contrast, in thermal narratives from Caldas da Imperatriz (Brazil), spontaneous talk does not focus on 'pains', 'illnesses' or 'problems', but the 'energy' of the water, the place (as 'nature'), the hotel, taking advantage of the visit, of doing a 'health treatment', of being able to 'go out' (considered therapeutic in this setting), 'rest', 'relax' and receiving 'energy' whether from the place itself, its waters, or as often happens, from Brother Hugolino.

According to Luzinete, aged 55, a retired bank employee, Kardecist spiritist and visitor to the thermal hotel for the last 15 years, an article in the *Folha de S. Paulo* newspaper about Caldas da Imperatriz made her curious to get to know the place. She describes her first visit to the spa remembering how the 'strength' and 'energy' of the water amazed her and how when she takes a bath she 'convinces herself' that she is receiving 'good energy'.

Through an analysis of the two categories – 'pain' and 'energy' – and the meanings the visitors attribute to treatment and use of the thermal water focused on the baths, the author identified explanatory models for this therapeutic practice that justify the carrying out of the fortnight or season, and reveal two concepts of the thermal visit: 'treating illness', 'treating health'.

The two models share the concept of thermal water as a 'natural' therapeutic agent due to its chemical ingredients or physical properties. Its therapeutic efficacy is ascribed equally to heat and the water's 'properties', as well as such 'elements' as 'salts', 'sulfur', 'radioactivity', 'minerals', and the absence of other 'products', namely 'chemicals' such as 'hypochlorites', for example. Since the thermal springs are seen as a product of nature, the air is also considered 'pure' and unpolluted. Moreover, the spa facility is seen as a 'family-like' environment.

In the Portuguese context, water is thought of as a 'natural medicine' due to its origins in 'nature', conceived as devoid of human intervention and therefore 'not harmful'. In contrast to medication, such as anti-inflammatories that 'are bad for the stomach', secondary effects are not attributed to it. Both doctors and spa-goers consider the water a 'natural medicine', although for different reasons: the former basing this on science, the latter basing it on the 'mysteries of water from nature' (Quintela 2001).

In Brazil, explanations for the efficacy of thermal water are not based merely on a particular element or substance it contains. Rather it is justified by the bodily experience the 'different water' causes, provoking sensations of 'lightness', 'well-being', 'relaxation', 'calm', 'energizing effect'.

As the author mentioned previously, there are various ways of consuming thermal water; however, here the author gives primacy to immersion or the 'bath'. In the Portuguese case this only has a therapeutic function and is thought of as a medicine and is administered according to standard, medically-regulated procedures. The baths (or 'treatments') described above, are scheduled, have a precise length, and a balneotherapy assistant administers them to the spa-goer who wears a bathing suit.

In Brazil, the baths have other purposes besides therapeutic, such as hygiene, relaxation, 'well-being', pleasure and 'energizing'. It is a time for taking care of hygiene, for healing, praying and pleasure. Various attributes are ascribed to the water: 'the water washes and cleans. It washes away everything that is bad. It cleanses the body. And the energy it transmits is really strong! And that energy comes from God, from a higher being, from above', guarantees Ana, a member of *União do Vegetal*, who sought the waters to 'harmonize herself'. The bathing ritual is what differentiates its purposes. Guests with a longer spa history affirm that 'the waters are mysterious', 'they are sacred', but the baths have to be 'done well'. At the hotel, everyone the author observed took at least two baths a day. And as a woman who has used the spa for 30 years explained:

> Listen, you have to know how to take a bath. I go in, I turn on the tap. I get in, sit down and let the jets spray my joints, mainly the places that hurt. You never put on soap when the water's turned off. They say that the soap eliminates the water's properties. Sometimes I use soap, but only in the morning. You turn off the water after taking off the soap, while you're inside. Me, when [the water] is overflowing, I submerse myself. The best thing is to submerse oneself and concentrate on that heat entering the body. That's when it feels good... I stay for 15 to 20 minutes.

Spa-goers to Portuguese and Brazilian spas have treatment rituals (and explanatory models for these) consisting primarily of baths: therapeutic bath length (15 to 20 minutes) and after-bath rest or relaxation. The author also encountered similar explanations for the baths' therapeutic efficacy – residing in the sweating effect the thermal water provokes, allowing 'toxins', 'the bad' to escape, since the 'good thing about the bath is the sweating'.

In these explanatory models, the therapeutic efficacy of the baths is attributed to the loss of 'sweat' and renewing the organism, a process in which the skin functions as an intermediary between the internal and external. The water 'penetrates' the 'body', the 'organism' via the skin, simultaneously expelling all excess substances considered unnecessary in an exchange process. But the 'mineral salts' and 'substances' the organism needs also enter through the skin. In both thermal contexts this is one of the reasons mentioned for not drying off the body with a towel afterwards since it would 'remove the substances'. In these conceptions, equilibrium – the basis for seeking thermal treatment – is achieved via this process of exchange. These explanations are based on humoral and naturalist theories that constitute the principles of thermal medicine (Porter 1990).

Similarly, the thermal bath is repeatedly represented as a bath for the water to penetrate the body, as opposed to a bath for 'cleansing' or 'hygiene' necessary for removing dirt from the body. Some distinguishing factors are bath length and the use of soap. In Portuguese spas soap is not used in the bathing area and the bath is not considered for 'hygiene'. Here the thermal water of the bath is used only medicinally, as the author has previously mentioned. It must also be noted, however, that at Hotel Caldas da Imperatriz (Brazil) some rooms do not have their own bathroom (*banheiro*, WC), so therefore, in this case, the thermal bath must also have a hygienic as well as therapeutic purpose.[11]

The ethnography reveals two concepts of thermal bathing practices anchored in two visions of the world. In the Portuguese context, the concept is based on notions of fatality and naturalization regarding health and illness that are attributed to the supernatural as well as to living conditions. The medicine is water, with treatment also including rest and consequently the interruption of daily activities. Although not explicitly, these views of thermal practice relate to theology of Catholic origins, which dictates that suffering should be endured as a God-given test for measuring levels of human resistance and faith. The idea that pains – namely from rheumatism – are chronic and therefore incurable and can only be treated, accentuates the notion that a state of suffering accompanies existence and must be endured. This does not mean they cannot be treated to alleviate the pain, as part of this process. Here, thermal medicine has a regulatory and care-taking role in a 'somatic society' (Turner 1996).

In the Brazilian context, the author finds the concept focuses on seeking well-being – highlighting the relationship between health and 'healthy society' and, accordingly, the need to unleash the 'energy' resource existing both in nature and in the individual. Therapeutic practices echo these explanations, interpenetrating religious and therapeutic domains, indivisible worlds that express holistic visions. It is also significant that medicalization does not emerge in the regulation of space, time and control and discipline of the body, allowing for idiosyncratic forms of therapeutic practice, one among other forms of therapeutic syncretism in the search for well-being. In this situation, healthy society is medicalized in the same way that some religious philosophies impose norms of individual behavior that intersect with collective ones. It is therefore understandable that therapeutic thermal practices in Caldas da Imperatriz are different from the Portuguese spas studied. Nevertheless, common principles remain in thermal medicine, the product of – naturalist, humoral, vitalistic – medical theories, and play off and intersect with other areas of life, creatively encompassing them to form new ways of achieving the ultimate goal of 'well-being'.

Ethnographic research revealed two concepts of thermal therapeutic practice: one concerned with 'alleviating' ailments (Portugal) and another seeking well-being (Brazil). One treats 'pains' while the other treats 'health'. In one case, 'pains' are mentioned and the stay is comparable to being in a hospital. In the other, 'energy' is mentioned and the stay represents an encounter with 'nature'. In the Portuguese context, discussing 'pains' is a form of treatment itself, 'alleviating' and lessening them and part of the therapeutic process. In the other, it is not necessary to speak of problems to 'treat [one's] health'. In this sense, it is possible to understand the different types of sociability observed in Portuguese and in Brazilian spas. In the first case, it focuses on the space and public spheres, resembling a communications exercise through which spa-goers share experiences of illness, suffering, pain, problems, in short, life. In the second case (Brazil), it focuses on private spaces and domains, and the individuality of these experiences in self-reflection is evident, even verbalized in some cases as a process of 'self-knowledge'. Here, illness, pain and problems are part of the private domain; the 'good things', the 'energy', the 'good *astral*' (vibes), belong to the public domain. To overcome and get over states of discomfort, *bricolage* experiments are carried out (Lévi-Strauss 1962) in which 'energy' mediates these states of discomfort and suffering, pleasure and entertainment. In contrast, in the Portuguese thermal context, the 'pains' (*dores*) and the illness are considered ontological states and an idiom central to a system of communication only explicable within this socio-cultural context.

Final considerations

Having analyzed the relationship between medicine and thermalism the author has observed that in Portuguese spas – due to the medicalization of thermal practices – bath use in particular is more disciplined and its therapeutic aspects heavily emphasized, thus justifying spa-goers' thermal visits (fortnightly) for illness and 'pains'. Nevertheless, this does not mean that following the 'baths' spa-goers do not enjoy recreation and leisure in spaces and times distinct from treatment. While doctors have the control to prescribe the correct and appropriate uses of mineral water, people visit spas also for leisure and recreation. But even when seeking leisure, people justify themselves by referring to the need for medical services.

In Brazil, the absence of a similar culture of medical hydrology meant that the 'medicalized' component of the spas never really developed. Without this, health regulations do not guide thermal practices in Caldas da Imperatriz. Nevertheless, guests have incorporated a medicalized discourse regarding daily practices of living and individual responsibility for health that is expressed in their rationale for using thermal water and the season to 'take care of health'. The therapeutic uses of the water can be defined as those of self-attention and self-prescription.

Thus, the author comprehends that in the Portuguese context the spas are sought to 'relieve pains' that go beyond 'rheumatic' ones. An annual thermal visit may interrupt the day-to-day conditions that cause this and, as some women say, 'this here is the best part of the entire year!', even if the 'baths' do not explicitly include a component of leisure as in the Brazilian spa. There, visitors use the thermal waters during the season to 'energize' themselves and 'return to the world' in better health, thus showing a holistic worldvision and perspective of health.

New legislation in both countries points to new forms and levels of medicalization and new configurations of the thermalism-medicine-tourism triad. This may signal greater control of thermal practices and spa settings in Brazil and a decrease of the same in Portugal, where the notion of 'well-being' was introduced and added to legislation regulating thermal activity. Only new studies will show what developments Brazilian legislative bodies will bring to these practices and reveal the relationship between this triad and the idiosyncrasies of this particular socio-cultural context.

The ethnographic comparison allowed for the study of the social, cultural and historical contexts that produce differing thermal experiences with distinct explanatory models regarding spa visits and practices in Portugal and Brazil. The author has found a certain social and cultural inversion of local conceptions about illness and health, such as 'pains' (*dores*), 'energy' (*energia*), and the association of 'problems' with notions of public and private.

'Pains' and 'energy' are not the only motives for seeking thermal treatment. They are also an idiom that reflects the center of a system of communication. Without this comparative dimension, it would not have been possible to become familiar with and understand the therapeutic and religious syncretism present in the practices and local explanations for thermal stays and treatment in the Brazilian context. Identifying the local categories of 'rheumatism', 'pains' and 'nerves', has made it possible to establish a dialogue with ethnographies conducted in other contexts (Good et al. 1994; Kleinman 1994; Pugh 2003; Jackson 2000; Low 1985; Shapiro 2003).

The comparison between the two contexts reveals that in the Portuguese cases medicine weakens the connection between therapy and religion. But in the Brazilian context, thermal practices are one of many possible alternatives for taking care of one's health, a fact that may be related to the diversity of alternatives found in the field of religion. As a consequence, the connection between the two fields, religion and medicine, permits the formation of a patchwork that mobilizes diverse social references and that suggests the following: if it is possible to choose the best of each system, why stick to only one? It is within this framework that thermalism in Brazil has developed – with medicalized thermal experiences of the nineteenth-century focusing on the 'curing' of illness reconfigured into apparently 'de-medicalized' practices focused on promoting well-being and the water's ability to 'cure' and 'energize'.

Acknowledgements

The author wishes to thank Jean Langdon, Cristiana Bastos and Renilda Barreto for their suggestions and Eva Graburn for translating and Catarina Mira for revising the paper.

Ethics: The places and institutions where the fieldwork was done did not have ethic research committees. However, ethnographic research and fieldwork ethics' principles were applied. A written explanation of the study was sent to all the institutions studied, asking for permission to do the fieldwork. To all the Spa-goers interviewed and observed the purpose of the study was explained and their anonymity was guaranteed. The names of interviewees are pseudonymous.

Funding: Science and Technology Foundation (FCT-Portugal) through PhD scholarship (SRH/BD/5240/2001) and projects coordinated by Cristiana Bastos – 'Water as a therapeutic agent: ethnography of spa practices in Portugal and Brazil' (CEAS, 2002–2004, POCTI/ANT/ 2001); 'From hot springs to spas: reconfiguration of a therapeutic practice' (CEAS, 2003–2006, POCTI/ANT/47274/2002). A version of this paper was presented in the session 'Healing Holidays' of the Society for Medical Anthropology meetings held at Yale University in 2009 and was part of the project 'The Circulation of Medical Knowledge' FCT - PTDC/ HCT//72143/2006.

Conflict of interest: none.

Notes

1. In Portugal, a doctor who practices at a spa must have a specialization in medical hydrology. Thermalism, as defined by Portuguese law (since 2004), is the 'use of mineral water and other agents for preventative, therapeutic, rehabilitative reasons and well-

being'. The Portuguese Association of Spas (ATP) has introduced new categories to this legislation: 'the classic thermalism segment' and the 'thermal and well-being segment'.

2. From the perspective of certain tourism and marketing studies, 'spa' refers to *'salut per la acqua'* or health through water, and is promoted as a consumer project. Today, the concept of spas is much wider and includes well-being and cosmetic practices that do not assume the existence of water, whether mineral, thermal or not. However, 'Spa' was the name of a Belgian setting that was very prominent in the European thermal scene beginning in the seventeenth-century. As Soye-Mitchell (1994) explains in her article about *villegiatura* in English cities during the eighteenth-century, in English, a city of waters is called a *spa*. This vocabulary appears in the language beginning in the seventeenth-century in the title of a short work celebrating the merits of a mineral spring discovered some years before, near Knaresborough in Yorkshire, which the author calls 'the English Spaw'. The spelling *spaw* survived up until the mid eighteenth-century. After being designated a so-called spring, the word *spa* applied precisely to the spring's location. Today it is called, for example, the Bath Spa or Leamington Spa (Soye-Mitchell 1994, 205). For origins of this vocabulary, see also Porter (1990), who associates it with the Belgian spring.

3. As a researcher on projects coordinated by Cristiana Bastos – 'Water as a therapeutic agent: ethnography of spa practices in Portugal and Brazil' (2002–2004) and 'From hot springs to spas: reconfiguration of a therapeutic practice' (2003–2006).

4. The Termas de São Pedro do Sul is considered one of the 'oldest' Portuguese spas, associated with the nation's beginnings (twelfth-century) and its founding monarch who frequented its waters. In recent decades, it has been the Portuguese spa most frequently visited (around 19,000 spa-goers per year) and currently has three times as many visitors as the establishment holding second place (Termas de Chaves, around 6500) in the Portuguese thermalism scene. Data collected in 1996–1997 as part of MA research, regarding thermalism and thermal experiences in Termas de São Pedro do Sul, is compared with the research presented here.

5. In 2003, this spa came in eighth place in a ranking of Portuguese spas, with 3500 spa-goers.

6. Medicalization is used here in the sense of Zola (1972), for whom medicine became one of the most powerful institutions of social control, incorporating the power traditionally exercised by law and religion.

7. In 1919, a decree was issued in Portugal establishing the bases for operating hydrology and climatology courses, also requiring clinical management to be present at thermal establishments. The Institute of Hydrology and Climatology was founded in Lisbon in 1919, in Porto in 1930 and in Coimbra in 1935, with the dual purpose of publicizing the therapeutic qualities of the waters and tourism at the respective spa settings.

8. *Vidáqua* is a shower that is taken in lying position while a massage is applied (it is known elsewhere as douche de Vichy); douche mouve is a circular shower with spray coming horizontally from all sides; Bertholaix is held in a small chamber where spa-goers sit in to steam the limbs and upper body; inhalotherapy entails nasal irrigation and aerosol treatment.

9. 'Tratar' may be literally translated into English as 'to treat', meaning to take care of but not necessarily to cure.

10. Brother Hugolino is a Franciscan monk of German descent who joined the *Conventinho do Espírito Santo* in Santo Amaro da Imperatriz in the 1980s, and who – linking parapsychology with religion – began administering 'cures with his hands'. Brother Hugolino appears in some of the regional tourist pamphlets – and currently on internet sites – as one of the places to visit on the 'religious tourism' circuit, just as Mother Paulina (the first saint from Brazil to be canonized) or the Grotto of Angelina, and visiting him symbolizes a high point on this touristic-religious and/or therapeutic tour. Visiting Brother Hugolino to receive a blessing is part of the thermal visit.

11. Taking an immersion 'bath' is generally not part of common daily practice for Brazilians, who rather shower.

References

Good, Mary-Jo, Paul Brodwin, and Byron Good, eds. 1994. *Pain as human experience. An anthropological perspective.* Berkeley: University of California Press.

Jackson, Jean E. 2000. *'Camp pain'. Talking with chronic pain patients.* Philadelphia: University of Pennsylvania Press.

Kleinman, Arthur. 1980. *Patients and healers in the context of culture. An exploration of the borderland between anthropology, medicine and psychiatry.* Berkeley: University of California Press.

Kleinman, Arthur. 1994. Pain and resistance: The delegitimation and relegitimation of local worlds. In *Pain as human experience. An anthropological perspective,* ed. Mary Jo Good, Paul Brodwin and Byron Good, 169–197. Berkeley: University of California Press.

Lévi-Strauss, Claude. 1962. *La pensée sauvage.* Paris: Plon.

Low, Setha M. 1985. Culturally interpreted symptoms or culture-bound syndromes: A cross-cultural review of nerves. *Social Science & Medicine* 21, no. 2: 187–96.

Mackaman, Douglas Peter. 1998. *Leisure settings. Bourgeois culture, medicine and the spa in modern France.* Chicago: Chicago University Press.

Porter, Roy. 1990. *Medical history of waters and spas.* London: Welcome Institute for the History of Medicine.

Pugh, Judy F. 2003. Concepts of arthritis in India's medical traditions: Ayurvedic and Unani perspectives. *Social Science & Medicine* 56, no. 2: 415–24.

Quintela, Maria Manuel. 1999. Curar e folgar: Etnografia das experiências termais nas Termas de São Pedro do Sul. Master Dissertation, ISCTE, Lisbon.

Quintela, Maria Manuel. 2001. Turismo e reumatismo: Etnografia de uma prática terapêutica nas Termas de São Pedro do Sul. *Etnográfica* 5, no. 2: 137–58.

Quintela, Maria Manuel. 2004. Práticas e saberes termais em Portugal e no Brasil. *História, Ciências, Saúde – Manguinhos* 11, supplement 1: 239–60.

Quintela, Maria Manuel. 2008. Águas que curam, águas que 'energizam': Etnografia das práticas terapêuticas termais em Portugal (Sulfúrea) e Brasil (Caldas da Imperatriz). PhD Dissertation, ICS – Universidade de Lisboa, Lisbon.

Shapiro, Hugh. 2003. How different are Western and Chinese medicine? The case of nerves. In *Medicine across cultures. History and practices of medicine in non-Western cultures,* ed. Helaine Selin, 351–72. Norwell: Kluwer Academic.

Smith, Valene, ed. 1989. *Hosts and guests. The anthropology of tourism.* Philadelphia: University of Pennsylvania Press.

Soye-Mitchell, Brigitte. 1994. La villégiature dans les villes d'eaux anglaises au XVIIIe siécle. In *2000 ans de thermalisme – actes du colloque tenu en Mars 1994 à Royat,* Dominique Jarrassé (org.), 205–214. Clémont-Ferrand: Publications de L'Institut d'Etudes du Massif Central.

Turner, Byron. 1996. *The body and society. Explorations in social theory.* London: Sage.

Weisz, George. 1995. *The medical mandarins. The French Academy of Medicine in the nineteenth and twentieth centuries.* Oxford: Oxford University Press.

Weisz, George. 2001. Spas, mineral waters, and hydrological science in twentieth-century France. *Isis* 92: 451–83.

Zola, Irving Kenneth. 1972. Medicine as an institution of social control. *Sociological Review* 20, no. 4: 170–85.

From sulphur to perfume: spa and SPA at Monchique, Algarve

Cristiana Bastos

Institute of Social Sciences, University of Lisbon, Portugal

In the thermal village of Monchique, Algarve, different streams of water-related knowledge and practices coexisted for centuries. Those waters were traditionally known as *águas santas* (holy waters) and believed to have redemptive healing powers. In the seventeenth century, the Catholic church took control of the place, refashioned the bathing rituals, developed infrastructures and provided assistance to the patients, granting free treatment to the poor. In the nineteenth century, the state replaced the church and imposed that treatments should be provided by professionals trained in the scientific principles of medical hydrology. Secular and scientific as they were, clinical logbooks still allowed for the account of patients that embodied miracle-like redemptive cures 'at the third bath'. People went to Monchique both for its magic and its medicine, bringing in the body ailments achieved in their lives of hard labour. They also went there for a socialising break while healing. From mendicants to rich landowners, coming mostly from the Algarve and neighbouring Alentejo, they crowded the place in summertime. In the twentieth century, as in other places in continental Europe, the spa evolved into a highly medicalised place that qualified for medical expenses reimbursements, which implied the eclipsing – at least from representation – of its leisure component. In the twenty-first century, a new trend of consumer-centred, market-based, post-water balneology with an emphasis on wellness and leisure reinvented the spa as place for lush and diversified consumption. This article argues that the seemingly contradictory systems (markets and medicine) coexist much in the same way that magic, religion and medicine coexisted in the old water sites. The new SPAs, rather than putting an end to the old spas, have enabled them to survive by reinventing thermal sites as places of attraction and leisure.

1. Redemption at the third bath

Pedro António, a 35 year old rope-maker from the fishing village of Portimão, Algarve, could only move about with the help of a pair of canes. With impaired mobility, a record of syphilis, and enduring rheumatic pain for at least one year, Pedro might have foreseen living the rest of his days as a disabled person or, to use the vernacular of the time, as an *entrevado* – a word that resounds both of 'paralysed' and of 'in the darkness'. And yet something happened in a late spring day of 1874

37

that changed the gloomy prospect: he started walking on his own, reportedly, after a series of three baths.

In the following weeks and months of the same year, a similar experience occurred to a tailor named João Brigadeiro, aged 24, from Lagos, Algarve, who traded his two canes for a simple umbrella, again after the third bath; and equally to the labourer Manuel José Passarinho, 34, also from Lagos, who dropped his supporting cane... after the third bath; and to Agostinho José, 30, labourer in Odemira, Alentejo; to Maria Henriques, 32, a housewife from São Brás, Algarve; and to José da Silva, 30, a labourer from Monchique, Algarve. All of them started walking unaided 'after the third bath'.

What sort of bathing was this? Where and when did it take place? What sort of people, knowledge, symbols, material objects and gestures were involved? While the reference to a biblical resuscitation 'at the third day' may lead us to think of a holy shrine, perhaps a holy well, or a religious ritual involving water, the fact of the matter is that these reports of spectacular, quasi-miraculous healing were registered within a very secular genre: nineteenth-century medical logbooks.

Pedro, João, Manuel, Agostinho, Maria and José were treated with the waters of *Caldas de Monchique* in the year 1874.[1] Each of them corresponds to one of the 749 line-entries that synthesise every patient's clinical history. The book was signed by the resident physician Francisco Lázaro Cortes and has survived until today. His comments on the redemptive 'third bath' appear as *fait divers* at the end of each line, just like 'got better', 'got cured', 'used *águas férreas*' (iron-rich waters from another spring in Monchique), or 'did not charge him for services provided at the spa' (referring to a doctor who stayed there), or 'came for the second time this year'. The redemptive 'third bath' was one more item in a log of personal and clinical data written about every person who received treatment.

Dr Francisco Lázaro Cortes and his logbook were novelties to Monchique. In 1872, the government had just established that the spa should have a resident physician to supervise the water treatments and register clinical data, so that science and professional clinical procedures replaced the current and perhaps inappropriate use of waters, solely based on traditional knowledge and religious good will.

There was a long history of healing acts and beliefs around the waters of Monchique. Like other springs and wells throughout Europe, those waters had been used for centuries as special, sacred, holy and redemptive of human suffering.[2] There are local archaeological remains from the Roman period (about 2000 years). There is notice that at least one notorious king, John II (1455–1495), used its waters.[3] However, also as in many other places, their users were mostly the anonymous peasants who left little material trace, but kept the beliefs and rituals alive throughout the ages. As with other things considered of the realm of magic and superstition, they were refashioned and re-styled by the Catholic church, which was hegemonic in Portugal since its beginning as a nation-state in the twelfth century.[4] In that process of disciplining the bodies, the gestures, the words and the worldviews of the peasantry, the church provided names of saints to the sources and pools; built chapels and shrines next to them; adapted the rituals and prayers used by the waters; provided charitable assistance to the poor and the indigent.

Catholic control over Monchique materialised most expressively in the seventeenth century. Through the orders of the bishops of Faro, Algarve, some basic shelters were built in 1649: one for bathing, one for lodging (with three beds and a chimney for cooking) and one for the servants and the poor. They were refashioned in 1672, but remained very basic. Major improvements came in 1691–1692, again via the orders of the bishops of Faro, who were granted the control of the place. The shelters were restored, an infirmary for the poor was added, a separate infirmary and dormitory for women was built in 1731. In 1752, 1780 and 1789 there were more improvements in the hospital, kitchen and baths, a mud pool was made, better accesses were opened, trees were planted and a physician from Lagos was brought to assist the poor (Acciaiuoli 1944, 169). In the early 1800s there were three pools for hydrotherapy, two of them named after saints – *São João de Deus,* with the capacity for 12 people, *Santa Teresa,* for up to six people, and, down the slope and large enough to hold up to 40 people, the pool of *Pancada* (literally, 'beating'), where the water fell from high up and hit the bodies like a strong shower (Tavares 1810; Soares 1835).

The church had to move out of the picture abruptly in 1834, when, in the aftermath of political upheavals, its estates all through the country, including the Algarve, were confiscated by the Portuguese government. For a few years, people used the waters of Monchique at their own risk, sometimes literally: with no supporting infrastructure, people would sometimes sleep under the trees, jeopardising the good effects of using the waters.

In 1840, the Algarve representative Mr Braklamy pleaded in the parliament for an urgent and rational intervention in Monchique. There was a wealth there, there seemed to be an exceptional healing power in its waters, one that had already cured thousands of paralytic and rheumatic patients in the past, and could eventually be used for respiratory diseases as well. This was too much to be left alone; it needed the professionalism of medicine and the universalism of science. There was also an underlying concern with the potential dangers of self-administration of mineral waters, a problem that in England had been compared to 'a sword in a madman's hands' by the advocates of the medicalisation of mineral waters (Harley 1990).

An increasingly secular state with a sympathy for medicine and science was to replace the church in the regulation of the access to water. There was a gap of inaction and neglect during the 1840s–1850s, a time when Charles Bonnet (1850) depicted the poor condition of Monchique and reported the indigence of his infrastructures, which were basically a building with two wings, separated by a dark and narrow corridor, having on one side the bath houses, chapel and kitchen, and little rooms for the bathers to rent, at the rate of 320 *réis* for 20 days. The government would soon intervene, sponsoring major renovations in 1862. By 1872 there was a regiment establishing the rules and the prices for taking the waters: 50 *reis* for a bath in the tub or in the small pool of *Santa Teresa,* 20 *reis* for a bath at the large *Pancada* pool, and 100 *reis* for a hygiene bath; those who had a certificate of poverty did not pay for the services. The improvements accounted for better ways of access, new infirmaries, and a permanent professional staff, which included two nurses of each sex, a clerk, laundry washers and janitors, and a resident physician, Francisco Lázaro Cortes, who supervised the treatments and the clinical record keeping.

In a curious way, amidst the standard banality of records about age, sex, birth, name, residence, profession, constitution, clinical background, previous conditions, prescriptions, results, Dr Cortes leaves a testimony about the persistence of a redemptive quality in the encounters of the suffering people and the reputedly holy waters. Some of the patients just dropped their canes and started walking... *at the third bath.*

2. A close look at the customers

Although there is no way to directly access the experience of those who walked after the third bath, it is possible to know a few things about them through the entries in the 1874 logbook – for instance, that all those six people were recent sufferers from the ailments or impairments that brought them to Monchique. Pedro Antonio's *reumatismo articular* (a broad definition for joint diseases) had been affecting him for a year, and was attributed to *arrefecimento*, or chilling, although syphilis is also listed in the column referring to pre-existing diseases. He arrived on 31 May and was prescribed a treatment of nine baths and 15 glasses of water. João, the 24-old tailor from Lagos, had been paralysed on his left side for about 4 months, his illness attributed to *apoplexia cerebral*, most likely what would be today referred as a stroke. He arrived on 4 June and was prescribed 15 baths and 22 glasses of water. Not only could he walk with the support of a simple umbrella after the third bath, but he left the place 'without the slightest sign of his disease'. Manuel, who walked in on a cane and dropped it after the third bath, suffered from *reumatismo articular* for the past nine months; in the past he had had malaria (*febres palustres*). He arrived on 14 June and was prescribed 15 baths and 15 glasses of water. Agostinho, the only one of this list of third-day-redemptions who was referred as 'poor' and as 'single', was a 30 year-old labourer from Odemira who suffered from generalized joint rheumatism (*reumatismo articular generalizado*) for the previous four months; like Manuel, his condition was attributed to 'chilling' (*arrefecimento*) and was prescribed 12 baths and 18 glasses of water after his arrival on 11 July. Maria, the 32-old housewife from São Brás, had suffered from sciatica over the period of a month with no apparent cause. She arrived on 31 July and was prescribed six baths, six showers and ten glasses of water. José, a local labourer who arrived towards the end of the season, on 16 September, had suffered for a month of what seemed an acute case of general joint rheumatism, probably related to his malarial condition (*febres palustres*). He was prescribed nine baths and 13 glasses of water.

Like Pedro, Maria, João, Manuel, Agostinho, and José, hundreds of men and women flocked to the waters of Monchique every year. Attendance was mostly seasonal, formally from May to September, but in fact starting in March–April and lasting to October–November (Figures 1 and 2). People came with rheumatic disorders, paraplegic conditions, impaired mobility, pain and discomfort. They came

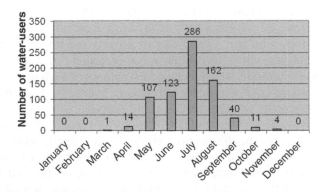

Figure 1. Monchique attendance, 1874: monthly frequency.

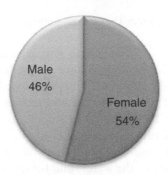

Figure 2. Monchique attendance, 1874: distribution by gender (346 men and boys; 402 women and girls).

from varied social backgrounds, with assorted ailments, and a common goal: to improve their condition via the use of the reputedly healing waters.

3. Monchique in a wider context

Bathing for wellness has been with humankind in many places and periods; sacred water holes exist around the world and major bathing cultures and architectures were developed at least under the Roman, Russian and Ottoman empires. The remnants of Roman water pipes, pools and extravagant bathhouses exist in sites that became spa-towns in later periods, as happened in Bath – the 'English Spa', a reference to the original 'Spa', a Belgian water site with a long tradition of curing and socialising. Bath catered not only to the illnesses but to the social needs of the eighteenth-century English gentry. Jane Austen provides a lively depiction of how families got together at Bath with the excuse of treating family members for gout, or simply without any medical excuse. Water drinking in the pump room punctuated a day filled with the activities of socialising, chatting, making friends, dressing up, parading, dining, dancing, establishing marriage alliances, developing the skills of conversation (Austen 1818; Hurley 2006).

That atmosphere was to decline in the following centuries, while, on the continent, spas flourished for a combination of reasons. Douglas Mackaman (1998) shows how the history of the French bourgeoisie and that of the modern spa are closely intertwined; vacationing according to the medicalised rhythms of the spa, but also to the sounds of ballroom dancing and casino gambling, was as much a constitutional part of the emerging class as their role in the production system. After a short period when the old spas were devalued for their associations with an aristocracy that had lost its high position in the French social structure, the reputation of the mineral water towns soon recuperated due both to the social needs of the emerging classes and to the developments of spa medicine. George Weisz (2001) argues that the development of medical hydrology and its institutionalisation as a respectful branch of medicine, its presence in medical curricula, and the lobbying power of its specialists, were crucial to maintain the centrality of water cures in France and achieve the one element that enabled, there and elsewhere, the longer survival of the old spa economy: the social security reimbursement of medically prescribed water cures.

Although a large number of French spas remained as austere in the nineteenth century as they had been in the renaissance (Brockliss 1990), the sophisticated architecture, landscaping and cultural activities developed in some of them provided a model for the development of some Portuguese *termas*, which aimed to attract the leisure-seeking classes, either from the still-existing local aristocracy or the emerging bourgeoisie. Vidago, Luso, Curia, Cucos, Caldas da Felgueira and others looked up to their French counterparts and tried to attract the fancy customers both on the basis of the therapeutic quality of the waters and the quality of leisure time one could spend there. Among the customers, some were *habitués* of the French, Italian and German spas, while others were new to the spa-culture. Old money and new money gathered in the palaces, grand hotels and casinos that were built around the *buvettes* (pump rooms) and bath houses of Luso, Vidago, Curia and other glamorous water springs. A liver condition, a troubled stomach, a rheumatic disorder, gout, pain, asthma, gynaecological ailments, neurasthenia, spleen, or recovery from the physical burdens of being in the colonies and other sites of 'tropical decay',[5] all were good motives for a period at the spa, where one could also bring along the family and socialise with those with similar motivations, tastes and social background. Spas became fashionable and desired experiences. In Ramalho Ortigão's (1875) account of spas & baths in Portugal, a suggestive illustration depicts a teenager indulging in self-pity for being left alone in the city while all her friends had gone to the waters.

Having a genuinely good time by the waters was not incompatible with being there for a healing purpose, as Ferreira (1995) and Quintela (1999, 2003) argued for later periods of intense medicalisation of the Portuguese spas, and Cátedra (2009) and Speier (2010) further argued for their Spanish and Czech counterparts. Going for a cure at a traditional spa, even if highly medicalised, was a way of taking a break from daily routines, be they the drudgeries of labour, the stresses of ownership, or the boredom of sheltered lives. To meet, mingle and play with the peers was at least as important to the spa-goers as treating the gout or sciatica that brought them there – or the effects of working a life at a mine in Asturias, as in the spa of Ledesma (Cátedra 2009). People have invented creative ways of combining leisure and treatment at the spa, from claiming enjoyment at the quasi-torture of some of the Forges treatments in the nineteenth century (Mackaman 1998) to gastronomic hedonism; as witnessed in the 1990s in some Portuguese spas by the author, and confirmed in the ethnography of S. Pedro do Sul (Quintela 1999), three and four-course meals with plenty of wine were more likely to be found than light food and water. Customers and restaurant managers alike argued that plenty of food and wine were a deserved compensation for the harshness endured at the water treatments.[6]

While some spas developed appropriate infrastructures for the needs of those who were more eager of entertainment than of treatments, others kept a more austere layout and a focus on their healing mission. Monchique in the late nineteenth century was somehow in between the two types. There were some improvements in the buildings that included a small 'casino', or a room to play cards and snooker, and there were pleasant views and airs to be enjoyed by the fashionable crowds seeking for status-promoting holidays at the spa. But Monchique, the 'narrow valley', with 'difficult accesses' (Bonnet 1850), distant from the trains – the railway did not reach the Algarve until 1899 – was also quite out of the way for the trendy urbanites. The clientele was mostly from the region, predominantly rural, reflecting the social structure in the countryside at the time.

4. Labour, class, pain and leisure in the south

In 1874, the clients of Monchique came mostly from the neighbouring Algarve villages and towns, from the nearby coast, and from the Alentejo. A good number came from Faro and Loulé, a few from the Eastern Algarve and one or two from Spanish Andalusia (Figure 3, Tables 1 and 2).

Among them, there were a few landowners, military officers and professionals that might use their time at the waters to build alliances and accomplish businesses, just like Austen's characters in Bath. There was a recreation room for playing cards and snooker (Ortigão 1875) and there were many outdoor locations to interact and socialise: by the water sources, under the trees of the valley or by the huge granite blocks that abound in the site. In the busier months, dozens of people gathered in Monchique at once, and there must have been a variety of forms of socialising. As in Vichy at the time (Mackaman 1998), this was not incompatible with the fact that some people suffered severe impairments, as it is reminded by the surviving wooden wheelchairs and litters kept in a small local museum at the spa.

Data from the logbooks indicate that the vast majority of those who went there had rheumatic diseases and other ailments of the bones and joints (63% to 73%, if sciatica and related disorders are included) and, to a lesser degree, skin, stomach and menstrual-related problems. Rich and poor, they had the chronic and acute versions of the omnipresent rheumatism.

Some of the clients appear as more pampered than others. Some women have a 'D.' before their name, for *Dona*; although it does not necessarily mean an aristocratic belonging, as would most likely be the case of a 'D.', for *Dom*, before a man's name,[7] *Dona* is a sign of distinction and deference, a marker of social status that sets them apart from common people and labourers. That was the case with the four ladies who arrived together on 13 May: D. Maria da Gloria, D. Anna Nunes d'Almeida, D. Maria Purificação Almeida, and D. Cecília Adelaide d'Almeida. They were all registered as single and as *domésticas*,[8] born in Pêra, Algarve, and residing there. They are likely to have been a group of land-owning close relatives from that small town who travelled together the few dozen miles between Pêra and Monchique. Only Anna, aged 34, had the ubiquitous *reumatismo articular* that affected most of the clients. She had had it for 4 months, the cause unknown. She was prescribed 13 baths and nine glasses of water. Maria da Gloria, aged 36, had 'herpes' for three years, and was prescribed seven general applications of water and 10 local applications, plus 13 glasses of water. Maria da Purificação, aged 24, had a lacrimal fistula for five years, probably caused by a 'lacrimal tumor'; she was prescribed nine general applications of water. Cecília Adelaide, 25, had dyspepsia for three years, attributed to 'lymphatism'. She was prescribed the ingestion of the iron-rich waters that came from a special spring in Monchique. All of them got better, except for Maria da Purificação, who neither improved nor worsened her eye condition. With no further data on this group, one can only speculate whether, were it not for Anna's rheumatism, the others would have ever made it to the spa.

Table 1. Residence of Monchique attendants, 1874.

Local: Monchique and surroundings	88
Algarve (5 km–25 km from Monchique)	320
Algarve (over 25 km from Monchique)	220
Alentejo	92
Spain	7
Others/unknown	21

Table 2. Occupation of Monchique attendants, 1874.

'Domestics'/'Housewives' (just the name)	236	31.6%
'Domestics'/'Ladies' (D.)	84	11.2%
Land owners	122	16.3%
Land labourers	75	10.0%
Crafts (weavers, tailors, charcoal-sellers, shoemakers, carpenters, cork cutters, rope makers, etc)	62	8.3%
Professions (public employees, physicians, nurses, business)	35	4.7%
Militaries	15	2.0%
Sailors	5	0.7%
Clergy	5	0.7%
Student	1	0.1%
Servants	23	3.1%
Beggars	11	1.4%
Unspecified	74	9.9%

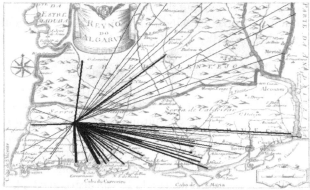
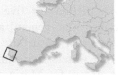

Figure 3. Geographic origin of Monchique attendants, 1874.

It is also possible that Anna's rheumatism was a solid enough motive to set in motion a project of taking the waters in Monchique, and once this was established, the other three women had no shortage of smaller afflictions that could use some virtuous water.

Other people were not as pampered as those four women and came to the spa with a life of hard labour behind their ailments. Some of their afflictions were a direct effect of working in agriculture or in the manual crafts they had as carpenters, weavers, spinners, tailors, sailors, miners, cork-cutters, rope-makers. Many among them had difficulties with their limbs and joints, probably the result of the repetitive movements they made in the exercise of their crafts. Others had secondary effects of malaria, which was quite prevalent among agriculture workers in the southern areas of Europe at the time. Others suffered the consequences of inadequate nutrition, poor housing, excessive exposure to the elements – the sea, the sun, the heat, the cold, the rain and drought.

About one fifth (155 in 749) of those who received treatment in Monchique in 1874 were classified as poor. In a tradition that had been established by the church, and followed by the secular state, they did not pay for their treatments. Nothing indicates that they were subject to a lesser treatment or considered a nuisance to the other customers, as reported by Mackaman (1998) for some of the French spas; nor is there evidence that the poor were segregated along with those who had leprosy and syphilis, as it happened in some older Portuguese spas.[9] But there were many other ways to materialise social stratification, such as with first-, second- and third-class bathing services. According to Sarzedas (1903), *São João de Deus* was the first-class bathing, and not a pool, but a service of individual bath tubs in private rooms, in a total of six; the smaller pool of *Santa Teresa* was the second class-bathing; and the larger pool of *Pancada* served as third class. It was most likely here that the poor immersed their bodies.

Among the poor there were mendicants, servants and other low-income or unemployed labourers. Almost all of them suffered from *reumatismo articular*, or 'joint rheumatism', corresponding to the broad spectrum encompassed by 'arthritis' in today's currency. Sometimes, arthritis appeared as a separate category, either unqualified, depicted as 'generalized', or 'muscular'. A number of the poor patients were diagnosed with sciatica. A few had other less common conditions for the time: Antonio Moniz, a 48-year old labourer from the town of Loulé, suffered from leprosy (*elephantiasis dos gregos*) on top of his arthritis. Manuel Maio, a 61-year old carpenter from Monchique, was paralysed on his right side (*hemiplesia direita*). José Gonçalves, a 15-year old boy from Lagos with no listed profession, had a 'painful ankylose' due to trauma. The waters brought him little relief and he left the spa using the same canes he came in with. The 3-year old child Antonio Simão, from the village of Algoz, Silves (Algarve), who was diagnosed as *paraplegico*, also remained unable to walk. Manuel Afonso, a labourer from Castro (Castro Verde, Alentejo), equally reported as *paraplegico*, kept moving around on his canes, and suffered from lower back pain. Ezequiel José, a labourer from Loulé who suffered from the joints and probably the bones (*osteite*) as a consequence of malaria, improved his condition after the treatments. Thereza Emilia, a 25 year-old weaver from Monchique, had experienced a radical improvement in the previous year, not yet subject to the rigorous statistics of a logbook. She had arrived to the spa in 1873 as an *entrevada* (disabled) and had left the place walking on her own, and she was still doing so when in 1874 she arrived for another round of baths.

5. The healing stench

As mentioned above, Caldas de Monchique stood somewhere in between the fancier Termas do Vidago, Curia, Luso and others, with their lush promenades, palace hotels and exquisite *buvettes*, and the Catholic thermal hospital better epitomised by Caldas da Rainha (Figure 4). Located in the central-western region of the country, about 100 km north of Lisbon, Caldas da Rainha (literally, 'The Queen's Hot Springs') was reputedly home to the first thermal hospital in the world (Mangorrinha 2000). It was built in the fifteenth century by order of a sensitive Queen Leonor (1458–1525) who, reportedly, had witnessed how the poor peasants sought to alleviate their pains and improve their arthritic and rheumatic conditions by bathing in the warm sulphurous springs and muddy pools that existed in the place. Legendary as this is, it reports that people used those waters to heal their body ailments. One of them was leprosy: in a royal edict from 1223, the Portuguese King Sancho II allowed the interns of a leprosarium from the city of Santarém to journey to the place that was chosen later as the site of the Thermal Hospital. There developed the town of Caldas da Rainha; there, also, the smell of sulphur lingered in the air.

Like those of Caldas da Rainha, the waters of Caldas de Monchique were rich in sulphur, and thus smelly, albeit to a lesser degree.[10] 'When entering the bath houses one immediately notices a sickening smell, mildly hepatic (*hepatico*) and suffocating', mentioned Dr Francisco Tavares in his 1810 general manual on Portuguese thermal waters. He noticed the white residue the water left in the pools and faucets; that the water was clear, but its taste sickening (*enjoativo*), 'with sparkles of iron'; and that

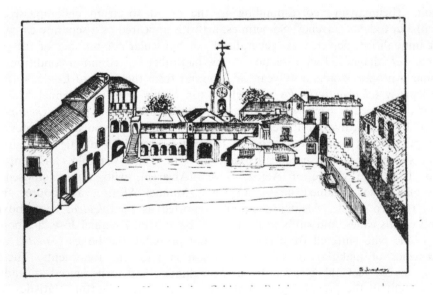

Figure 4. Caldas da Rainha, Portugal, sixteenth century.

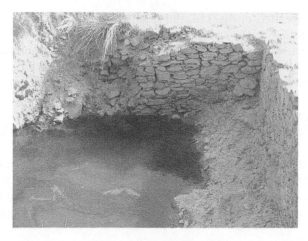

Figure 5. Rudimentary pool of sulphur water, out in the wild. © Leonor Areal.

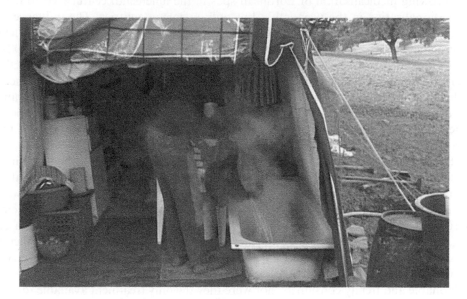

Figure 6. Self-catering, camping spa. © Leonor Areal.

after it cooled, the taste and smell would disappear, making the water totally suitable for drinking and cooking (Tavares 1810).

Sulphur, or the healing stench: its resemblance to hell, often reported by those who reflected upon its features, helped people out of the hell-like experience of bodily pain and impairment. The intense, 'sulphurous', rotten-egg smell of some waters is popularly associated with their healing powers. This was a belief widely shared across time and space, as Harley (1990) notes in his analysis of eighteenth- and nineteenth-century British manuals on mineral waters; in a 1803 treatise on the waters of Cheltenham, Dr. Thomas Jameson referred that 'if they had no bad taste nor smell, the patients would have no confidence in their virtues' (Harley 1990: 52).

Whether appreciated or disliked, the smell persists in the air and remains in the skin, hair and clothes of the spa-goers; some claim that after a time of disliking it, they end up addictively craving for it. The smell also lingers around the ponds which, out in the wild, still attract people to take the waters at their own risk (Figures 5 and 6); people that camp next to smelly water ponds with no other infrastructure than the equipment they brought to heat the water and bathe; people that have their own views and interpretations for the reasons behind the powers of sulphur water – be it the 'energy achieved from the rocks' or its deeper 'connections to the center of the earth'.[11]

In codified manuals, like the *Aquilégio Medicinal*, sulphur appears in association to Monchique's virtues: 'plenty of water, with sulphur, with great power (*virtudes*) for curing paralyses, stupor, all nerve conditions, and also stomach debilities, seizures, and other things that sulphur baths are good for' (Henriques 1726).

6. From sulphur to perfume

The growing medicalisation of European spas in the nineteenth century led to their institutionalisation in the twentieth – but only in some countries. The influence of medical hydrologists in making the field respectable and legitimate, and their treatments qualifying for reimbursement, well identified by George Weisz (2001) for France, had no counterpart in the British Isles. British spas declined while the French, German and also Portuguese ones flourished and their credibility enhanced – plus their use became routine to the many who believed in them, enjoyed them, and eventually used them for reimbursable medical holidays, reinforcing the 'medical' experience and talking more expressively of the painful side of it rather than of the pleasures associated with it.

Progressively, only the people on prescription went to the water springs. Excessive medicalisation of the Portuguese spas pushed the 'lure of the water' (Corbin 1988) towards the shores. Many places developed along the coastline with the new trend: Estoril and Cascais, close to Lisbon; the fishing shores of Ericeira (Jerónimo 2003) and Nazaré, further north, or Sesimbra, to the south; Figueira da Foz, next to Coimbra; the colder northern coast next to Oporto and the Galician coast of Vigo; and, at a later time, the golden cliffs and sunny beaches of the Algarve.

By the 1960s–1970s, Portuguese spas were no longer the first choice for fashionable and trendy consumers, nor were they the only treatment available for the sufferers of rheumatic diseases. Still, many people continued to visit them for treatment, and would not give up on having a good time while there (Ferreira 1995; Quintela 1999). They were mostly the ageing folks who preferred sharing the spa season (*temporada*) with their peers rather than going to the beach with younger family members, or who preferred submitting themselves to the time-consuming spa treatments rather than using pharmaceutical drugs, which they also dismissed either as useless or as having vicious side effects. They enjoyed meeting their partners in rheumatism and talking about their conditions, resembling an *avant-la-lettre* patient support group for people who often had no other choice for vacation and leisure than to take sick leave and receive medically prescribed treatments.

In sum, towards the end of the twentieth century, most Portuguese spas catered to an ageing and highly medicalised clientele. *Termas* seemed in frank decline, until a new trend began: the slow de-medicalisation of the spa and its reinvention as SPA.

In general terms, the 'new spas', or SPAs, only partially resemble the older ones. Some emerged in the location of the old spas, benefiting from their reputation, existing travel routes and material resources that include exquisite architecture and prime landscape, not to mention what had once been central, the warm springs. In other cases, the new SPAs have appeared as subsections of old spas, as an extension of their products and services. Other times, SPAs have been built anew, whether or not around classified mineral water springs. The word 'SPA' is sometimes used as qualifier and added to a hotel's name, as the words 'palace' or 'grand' were in the past.

SPA invented itself as an acronym from the Roman-Latin etymology: 'Sanitas Per Acqua'. Not the town of Spa, in Belgium, a reminder of the sleepy old *villes thermales* that came alive every season with flocks of ailing *curistes* with numerous family members and protégées in tow, ready to socialise and make do with the rituals of assessing one's place in society.

The SPA is not about illness or disease: it presents itself as of health and well-being. The SPA is not sponsored by the state or by medical hydrology. Its attendance does not require a medical prescription, or the cultural capital of a family *habitus*; it requires money – or credit – and a lifestyle. The SPA is not about repeating an old formula supported by a branch of medicine and scrupulously followed by clients/patients. The SPA-goers like the diversification of SPA products and services; they like variety, innovation, choice; thcy likc to feel free from the rules and regulations that structured attendance at the medicalised old spas. They like to be clients, not patients; they are consumers, not sick people. They carry credit cards and cash, not diseases. They want to purchase scented baths and exotic massages, not medical treatments. They want to decide whether to take a bath or ten, rather than follow the mandatory two or three weeks of daily treatments recommended by medical hydrology, sanctioned by commonsense, prescribed by resident clinicians and required by health insurance for reimbursement.

The new SPA does not really require the existence of thermal water, and sometimes there is no need of water other than to wash the body after coating it with extravagant products such as chocolate, grapes, coffee beans, lotions, oils, all amidst fancy massages, warm stones, crystal therapies, walks in the woods, meditation, mountain biking, gourmet food sampling and aromatherapy. In the new SPA, there is a clear preference for the flowery and pleasurable scents of perfumes, while the stench of sulphur, a reminder of the painful endurance of old style treatments, is – if it ever is around – carefully kept away from the wellness rooms.

7. Monchique, spa and SPA

By the beginning of the twenty-first century, and after a history of different managements, decay and reconstructions, Caldas de Monchique reinvented itself as a modern spa-town, anticipating a trend that spread rapidly to most other locations as well. While, in the past, people visited the place for heavily ritualised programmes of thermal water-bathing, showering, inhaling, or drinking, all meant to heal and cure, today they mostly go there for self-designed programmes that may include water drinking, but also wine, coffee, tea, beer and liquor tasting; it may include bathing in mineral water, but at their pleasure and leisure, in pools or Jacuzzi-powered bathtubs, combined with immersions in fashionable SPA products ranging from chocolate to wine grapes and seeds, milky lotions and exotic balms. Water is no longer drunk at the *buvette*, still warm and smelly from the spring, and in the exact amount prescribed. Now, water may be consumed cold from odourless dispensers, at any time and any place for free, or purchased and carried home in bottles of *Água de Monchique* or in its neatly designed new product, the 'chic' water.

Is that all Monchique has today, its miracles turned ancient myths? Has the SPA erased the medical spa, made it past history, bringing back the religious cult of nature and its elements in the form of a hedonist celebration of the senses backed by a cash-and-credit economy? Not really. Although less visible, having moved from the centre to the side of the place, the medical spa still exists and a significant number of patients attend it every year. In 2008, there were 621 people (230 men and 391 women) who went there for treatment, a number not too far from the 749 visits in 1874.

Today, however, people come from further away; a large number reside in Lisbon, although their families may come from the Algarve and Alentejo. As in the past, they come in the summer, but peak attendance is in September, not, as in the past, July. They come mostly for muscular-skeletal (*musculo-esqueléticas*) disorders, still the general category for the same variety of disorders called *reumatismo* in the past. They come also to treat their throat and their respiratory disorders and, to a lesser degree, their stomach ailments. While the majority does not experience immediate results (16.4% declare improvement, while 83.6% declare that they remained the same), a large majority improve their condition in the long run: 31% report 'mild improvement', 48.4% report 'improvement', and 15% report 'strong improvement'.[12]

While no longer 'at the third bath', and no longer as in a miracle, people still claim that the waters of Monchique can heal them.

8. Conclusion: has the SPA put an end to the medical spa?

In summary, the SPA has not replaced or put an end to the old spa. Instead, the argument of this article is that the SPA has enabled the old spa to survive, by reinventing thermal sites as places of attraction, leisure, and consumption. In the older version, spas were mostly about healing, and the church was keen to administer the reputed miracles of their waters. In the nineteenth century, the trend of medicalisation attracted a growing number of clients who enjoyed their disciplined, medically-supervised vacations as well as the accompanying glamour. In the twentieth century, as spa medicalisation became stricter, leisure-seeking clients turned elsewhere, either to the beach, the mountains, radical sports, gambling, eco-travel, or other assorted products invented by the tourist industry. Towards the end of the twentieth century, spas were in serious decline and many people foresaw their total extinction. And yet, in the twenty-first century, spas have reinvented themselves as SPAs, introducing leisure as a product and flexible consumption as a mandate. But, contrary to some predictions, the new SPAs coexist well with the old spas. At least, this is the case in Monchique, which continues to cater to a number of visitors that, in the end, differs little from the seven hundred plus who sought its waters in the year 1874.

Acknowledgements/Funding

Research for this paper was funded by the projects *Empires, centers and provinces: the circulation of medical knowledge* (FCT-PTDC/HCT/72143/2006), and *Das termas aos Spas: reconfigurações de uma prática terapêutica* (FCT- POCTI/ANT/47274/2002). The author thanks Antonio Perestrelo de Matos and Maria Manuel Quintela, who were part of the research team that surveyed virtually all water springs in continental Portugal, and to Frederico Rivera and Jorge Rivera, who volunteered in the survey with enthusiasm. Further thanks go to Leonor Areal for the photographs, to Alexandra Baixinho for maps, to the Monchique Spa Director Tiago Martins Barata, who made access to sources an easy and enjoyable task, and to the many anonymous users of mineral waters that throughout the country shared with the team their views and perspectives. The author would also like to acknowledge the insightful, generous and useful comments and suggestions of the anonymous reviewers of this article.

Ethics committee requirements: research draws on data from the nineteenth century. No human subjects were involved in experiences. The person in Figure 6 consented in being photographed.

Conflict of interest: none

Notes

1. *Caldas*, like *termas*, stands for warm water springs, and 'Monchique' (reportedly from the Arabic names for 'sacred mountain') refers to the mountains where they are located, in the western Algarve, southern Portugal. *Caldas de Monchique* and the nearby town of the same name are about 20 km off the southern shore (Alvor, Lagos), 25 km off the western shore (Aljezur), and 10 km off the dividing line with the Alentejo province (County of Odemira). Those mountains result from a granite-sienite surfacing amidst a mostly schist and limestone geology. As in northern Portugal, the warm sulphur springs appear most often along with the granite. The data hereby presented come from the clinical logbook started in 1874, which is kept in good condition and belongs to the historical collection preserved at the Monchique estate.
2. For example, Logan (1981), Bord (2006, 2008); while literature on pre-historic medicine and ethnomedical systems of knowledge has focused primarily on the therapeutic use of plants and disregarded the role of water-based healing, the literature on ancient bathing has focused primarily on leisure, hygiene and social regulation (e.g. Jackson 1990), leaving thus unattended the area of pre/historic or ancient water cures.
3. Reputedly poisoned by his enemies, John sought treatment in the Monchique, but not even those waters were able to rescue him. Ill-fated King Sebastian (1554–1578) is also reported to have passed by Monchique on his way to the fatal battle of Alcacer Kibir (Morocco). Other mineral springs had more auspicious encounters with royalty: the waters of São Pedro do Sul treated Afonso Henriques' (1111–1185) war fractures; Caldas da Rainha, (Queen's spa) owed its hospital, its name and its existence to the grace of Queen Leonor (1458–1525); in Brazil, Caldas da Imperatriz (Empress' spa) mimicked that name while paying homage to the visit of the recently empowered empress Leopoldina (1797–1826), wife of the first monarch of Brazil, Emperor Pedro.
4. Dating back to 1143, Portuguese independence was, since its beginning, closely associated with Christianity: northern crusade knights got involved in local Iberian disputes and in the 'reconquest' of the southern lands from the Muslim rule. Rome supported the new Christian kingdom, which kept some degree of religious tolerance towards its Jewish and Muslims communities until the early sixteenth century, when non-Christians were expelled, slaughtered or converted by force.
5. Portuguese colonial officers were often prescribed spa treatments back home in order to recover their balance and health. There are several references to leaves of absence in Portuguese colonial records that included temporary spa treatments. To my knowledge,

though, there were no attempts of turning the water springs located in the colonies into spas, as Eric T. Jennings (2006) so thoroughly describes for the French empire.

6. Fieldwork in the 2000s showed that the emergence of wellness SPAs helped to open a niche for lighter foods, timidly making room among the hedonistically heavy cuisine that pervades in most places.

7. This is valid for the Portuguese language, where the use of *Dom* is mostly reserved, although not exclusively, for aristocracy and high clergy, as opposed to Spanish, where *Don* is applied to a wide number of gentlemen.

8. *Doméstica*, literally 'from home', is most often translated as 'housewife', but it really does not mean that they were part of a husband-and-wife couple. The term was used to refer to the women who did not work outside the home, either poor or rich. Although vague, the classification stands in the way for a better understanding of the social stratification of the female population of water users.

9. Evidence was collected in the course of the project *Das termas aos spas* and is published on the site www.aguas.ics.ul.pt.

10. It is not the sulphur in itself that has the smell, but its dioxide, which resembles the unpleasant odour of rotten eggs. Some of the hot springs of the granitic lands of Northern Portugal, such as São Pedro do Sul, Caldas da Felgueira, Alcafache, etc, have a smell that is far more intense than that of Monchique, which can hardly be noticed today.

11. In the course of fieldwork in rural Portugal in 2003–2004, the research team found a number of people taking the waters in the most precarious conditions, in quasi-barracks or out in the wild, either self-catering or using very basic shelters where the water was supplied by ad hoc assistants who lived nearby or happened to own the shelter (Bastos 2004, 2006).

12. All data refer to the clinical report for the 2008 thermal season of Caldas de Monchique, signed by the clinical director Dr Estela Maria Quintino Avelar de Castro. The author is very grateful to Tiago Martins Barata and Claudia Vilela, from the spa management, for kindly providing the data.

References

Acciaiuoli, Luís de Meneses. 1944. *Águas de Portugal: minerais e de mesa: história e bibliografia*. Lisboa: Direcção Geral de Minas/Soc. Tipográfica, Vol. IV.

Austen, Jane. 1818. *Northanger Abbey*. London: John Murray.

Bastos, Cristiana. 2004. A cura pelas águas: estado da questão, tendências históricas e notas etnográficas. Paper delivered at the seminar *A cura pelas águas em portugal: estudos antropológicos, históricos e patrimoniais,* Termas do Luso, 17–18 July.

Bastos, Cristiana. 2006. Das Termas aos 'Spas': reconfigurações de uma prática terapêutica. http://www.aguas.ics.ul.pt/docs/dinamicas.pdf

Bonnet, Charles. 1850. *Algarve (Portugal): description géographique et géologique de cette province*. Lisbonne: Typ. de la Acad. Royale des Sciences.

Bord, Janet. 2006. *Cures and curses: Ritual and cult at Holly Well*. Loughborough: Heart of Albion Press.

Bord, Janet. 2008. *Holy wells in Britain: A guide*. Loughborough: Heart of Albion Press.

Brockliss, L.W. 1990. The development of the spa in seventeenth-century France. *Medical History Supplement*, no. 10: 23–47.

Cátedra Tomás, Maria. 2009. El agua que cura/Healing Waters. *Revista de Dialectología y Tradiciones Populares* LXIV, no. 1: 177–210.

Corbin, Alain. 1988. *Le territoire du vide: L'Occident et le désir du rivage, 1750-1840*. Paris: Aubier.

Ferreira, Claudino. 1995. Estilo de vida, práticas e representações sociais dos termalistas. O caso da Curia. *Revista Crítica de Ciências Sociais* 43: 93–122.

Harley, David. 1990. A sword in a madman's hand: Professional opposition to popular consumption in the waters literature of Southern England and the Midlands, 1570–1870. *Medical History*, Supplement 10: 48–55.

Henriques, Francisco da Fonseca. 1726. *Aquilégio Medicinal...*, Lisboa: Oficina da Música.

Hurley, Alison E. 2006. A conversation of their own: Watering-place correspondence among the bluestockings. *Eighteenth-Century Studies* 40, no. 1: 1–21.

Jackson, R. 1990. Waters and spas in the classical world. *Medical History Supplement*, no. 10: 1–13.

Jennings, Eric T. 2006. *Curing the colonizers: Hydrotherapy, climatology, and French colonial spas*. Durham: Duke University Press.

Jerónimo, Rita. 2003. Banhistas e Banheiros: Reconfiguração Identitária na Praia da Ericeira. *Etnográfica* 7, no. 1: 159–69.

Logan, Patrick. 1981. *The Holy wells of Ireland*. Ireland: Colin Smythe.

Mackaman, Douglas Peter. 1998. *Leisure settings: Bourgeois culture, medicine, and the spa in Modern France*. Chicago: University of Chicago Press.

Mangorrinha, Jorge. 2000. *O lugar das termas: património e desenvolvimento regional: as estâncias termais da Região Oeste*. Lisboa: Livros Horizonte.

Ortigão, Ramalho. 1875. *Banhos de caldas e águas mineraes*. Porto: Magalhäes & Moniz.

Quintela, Maria Manuel. 1999. *Entre Curar e Folgar: etnografia das termas de S Pedro do Sul*. Tese de Mestrado. Lisboa: ISCTE.

Quintela, Maria Manuel. 2003. Banhos que Curam: Práticas Termais em Portugal e no Brasil. *Etnográfica* 7, no. 1: 171–85.

Sarzedas, J.A.R. Tenreiro. 1903. *Relatório sobre a inspecção médica às águas mineraes e suas estancias em 1902*. Lisboa: Imprensa Nacional.

Soares, Alexandre Augusto de Oliveira. 1835. *Considerações fysiologico-praticas sobre a medicina cutânea*. Lisboa: Typ. da Academia Real das Sciencias.

Speier, Amy. 2011. Health tourism in a Czech spa. *Anthropology and Medicine* 18, no. 1: 55–66.

Tavares, Francisco. 1810. *Instrucções e cautelas practicas sobre a natureza, diferentes especies, virtudes em geral, e uso legitimo das águas mineraes, principalmente de Caldas*. Coimbra: Real Impr. da Universidade.

Weisz, George. 2001. Spas, mineral waters and hydrological science in twentieth-century France. *Isis* 92, no. 3: 451–83.

Health tourism in a Czech health spa

Amy R. Speier

Department of Anthropology, Eckerd College, St. Petersburg, Florida, USA

This paper is about the changing shape of health tourism in a Czech spa town. The research focuses on balneotherapy as a traditional Czech healing technique, which involves complex drinking and bathing therapies, as it is increasingly being incorporated into the development of a Czech health tourism industry. Today, the health tourism industry in Mariánské Lázně is attempting to 'harmoniously' combine three elements – balneology, travel and business activities. One detects subtle shifts and consequent incongruities as doctors struggle for control over the medical portion of spa hotels. At the same time, marketing groups are creating new packages for a general clientele, and the implementation of these new packages de-medicalizes balneotherapy. Related to the issue of the doctor's authority in the spa, the changes occurring with the privatization of tourism entails the entrance of 'tourists' to Mariánské Lázně who are not necessarily seeking spa treatment but who are still staying at spa hotels. There is a general consensus among spa doctors and employees that balneotherapy has become commodified. Thus, while balneotherapy remains a traditional form of therapy, the commercial context in which it exists has created a new form of health tourism.

Introduction

One year of ethnographic research on health tourism[1] took place in Mariánské Lázně, a Western Bohemian town with abundant sources of natural mineral springs. Mariánské Lázně has also been called Marienbad – a name still used by its German clientele. During the first four months of the research, methodology included participant-observation, informal and formal interviews at five different tourism agencies. Each agency arranged travel or spa services for hotel guests, some strictly catered to German tourists seeking information about the town, souvenirs, concert tickets, or excursions to outlying areas. During the summer tourist season, methodology entailed an additional four months of participant observation and interviews in five different spa hotels that administered balneotherapy. Access was granted to observe employees administer the full range of treatments to guests. The anthropologist often donned the obligatory white uniform as she talked to Czech health workers and guests. During the final phase of research, formal interviews were conducted with spa doctors and patient tourists. The German patient tourists required the aid of a translator.

Mariánské Lázně boasts a population of 14,000, which nearly doubles in the summer as the tourist season begins. High elevation accounts for the relatively clean, crisp air. *Hlavní Ulice*, or Main Street, runs along the town, which is divided into two parts: the lower part is a residential area, and as one ascends the hill, large, yellow hotels and spas in neo-classical, neo-renaissance, and neo-baroque architectural styles sit enveloped by forested mountains. Centrally located parks designed by the famous Czech landscape architect Skalník lead people to the main colonnade. Greenery envelops the mineral springs that are protected by smaller colonnade buildings throughout the town.

A Czech spa resembles traditional 'watering places' that have sources of mineral or thermal springs. The term *lázně*, or spa, in the Czech Republic denotes a place that administers balneotherapy, or treatments that use natural sources such as mineral waters, gas that comes from the earth, mud or peat bogs. People visit Czech spas for an average of three weeks and undergo various treatments that are prescribed by the spa doctor.

The research focuses on balneotherapy as a traditional Czech healing technique, which involves complex drinking and bathing therapies, as it is increasingly being incorporated into the development of a Czech health tourism industry. In the post-socialist period, the Czech economy relies heavily on tourism as a source of revenue, and spa towns are the second most popular attraction after Prague. According to the Czech Tourism website, nearly 7 million foreign tourists visited the country in 2008.

This paper examines the ways in which the health tourism industry of Mariánské Lázně is attempting to 'harmoniously' combine three elements: balneology, travel, and business. While health tourism has always been the main industry in Mariánské Lázně, the new globalized realm of spa business has created certain incongruities as doctors struggle for control over health regimens that are increasingly marketed and packaged by marketing corporations.

History

Historians refer to health spas as one of the earliest travel destination sites, since people began to travel under doctors' prescriptions (Aron 1999). The end of the nineteenth century and the beginning of the twentieth is considered to be the period of great prosperity for Western Bohemian spas. In Mariánské Lázně, Habsburg officials commanded the construction of several hotels and facilities that would contain the springs that patients sought out for their medically prescribed, regimented cures. At this time, healing waters were mainly reserved for aristocrats and the upper classes. The town offered a social setting for leisure as well as an elitist form of healing.

After the Second World War, spas were nationalized and set aside for domestic use and controlled by the state. The state proclaimed it was restoring balneotherapy to the masses through nationalization (Jirásek 1979). By the mid 1960s and the 1970s, most workers visited Mariánské Lázně for health treatments funded by their National Insurance (Nepustil 1949; Jirásek 1979; Carter 1991). Thus, balneotherapy was authorized as legitimate medicine by the socialist regime. In fact, the state intended to remodel these large healing sources primarily as medical institutions, rather than as elite resorts (Prerovský 1957).

Spas were also open to particular trade unions (see also Noack 2006). Trade unions took over half of the hotels. The majority of guests were 'recreants' who were sent by their unions – mainly ROH – *Revoluční Odborové Hnutí*. Recreants were provided with free accommodations in spa hotels as incentives or rewards for labor. The anthropologist's landlord, Petr, explained, 'They had special worker or labor unions who got to go to Mariánské Lázně for a free week, and it was for recreants. They worked hard and then they came to rest.' While they stayed, they could enjoy nights of dancing and drinking, in addition to the relaxing treatments offered at the spas. Thus, the state blended standard balneological medicine and recreation in order to maintain worker productivity. Leisure was understood to improve the standard of living (Carter 1991).

The fact that balneotherapy was legitimate state medicine explains why it has remained a central branch of rehabilitative medicine in the Czech Republic today. The socialist state set up various institutions for research and study that were aimed at proving the scientific basis of balneotherapy. The key importance of spa medicine was that it was geared toward rehabilitating citizens and restoring their ability to work.

Since the end of socialism, Mariánské Lázně is trying to regain its reputation as a vacation and health resort for people from all over the world. One corporation, Lečebné Lázně, has a monopoly and owns all of the spas. There are approximately 30 hotels that offer treatment packages as well, and new ones open annually. Private owners of spas and hotels are trying to redefine the socialist synthesis of health and leisure in specific ways that are explicitly oriented toward market-based consumption rather than production.

Balneotherapy

Balneotherapy entails a complex range of therapeutic procedures involving mineral spring water, peloids, and natural gases. Both peat and mud rank as peloids, and the particular peloid used in Mariánské Lázně is *slatina*. Mineral waters of various chemical components are professed to heal chronic diseases, some of which are diseases of the digestive tract; metabolic disorders; illnesses of the respiratory system; disorders of the locomotor system and the kidneys and urinary tract. These natural elements help renew a person because of their strength, and the title *lázně* is only applied to towns locally rich in natural resources. Traditional treatments entail four full regimented weeks of strict diet, exercise and fitness programs, complex therapies such as hydrotherapy, gas injections, electrotherapy, inhalation, and paraffin packs.

Mariánské Lázně is surrounded by kilometers of mountains covered by forests. Owing to the high elevation, the air is said to be healthier. Nature, in terms of balneotherapy as well as the 'natural' environment of the spa town, is spoken of as a healing agent. Nature is often personified as generous and healing. Nature helps people regenerate, using the force of its healing powers. The parks, which dot the landscape of the spa town, are referred to as the 'jewels' of Mariánské Lázně, and they are integrated into the walking cures for patients.

The basis of Mariánské Lázně's fame is its abundance of different cold, acidulous mineral waters. Of the 40 mineral waters of Mariánské Lázně, only eight or so are accorded healing properties that are part of a doctor's prescription. The springs that are used in medical prescriptions have been funneled to a central location on the colonnade for spa guests. The mineral waters that are used for treatment have been proclaimed 'healthy' by the ministry of health, based on scientific and hygienic criteria. Waters are the basis for the drinking cure, for which each patient drinks two cups before every meal. Waters are used for the treatment of digestive tract or urinary tract disorders. Mineral waters are also used for mineral baths.

Mariánské Lázně is the only spa that treats kidney diseases in the Czech Republic, and this is listed as its main indication. Most illnesses that are indicated for balneotherapy are chronic. A doctor explained,

> Balneotherapy functions according to different diagnoses. We have natural procedures that help circulation, and regeneration of the tissues. For the kidney diseases is the drinking treatment. For movement, for arthritis, is to lessen the pain they have with balneotherapy. With arthritis, is to improve movement. We want to stabilize [the patient] so an acute attack will not be often. We want to reinforce muscles through active procedures.

Improved circulation is part of the analgesic effect of nearly every procedure offered. A tour guide, Ilona, explained it in her own terms, 'A lot of the treatments are for blood circulation and I think the quickened blood circulation speeds up healing and the blood takes away the bad stuff.' In response to the question of why circulation was so important, one doctor said, 'Because when the body doesn't have oxygen the muscles wither and shrink and go to hell.' Oxygen travels to the heart, the lower limbs, and to bodily tissues. Spa doctors and assistants considered circulation as nutrition for the body. This, they said, explains why patient tourists feel better after their procedures. One German man spoke for himself and his wife:

> We are on treatment at New Spa...We are here for two weeks...we have the massage, the gas injections, the mineral bath, the gas pack, the electrotherapy...I already feel one hundred percent better, because of the massage mainly. We are drinking Rudolf and Caroline according to doctor's recommendation.

Just as balneotherapy treats the body as a whole, the procedures for a patient all work as a complex whole – it is not just one particular procedure that helps. The treatment schedules are said to be individualized for each patient. In addition to the drinking cure, most patient tourists have two to three procedures a day, which last approximately 20 to 30 minutes each. Older patients usually tire from having as few as two or three a day.

According to the guests undergoing spa treatments, procedures fall under the 'pleasant' or 'unpleasant' categories. There are pleasant procedures, such as massages, and unpleasant procedures, which are few, but include gas injections, which are subcutaneous injections of Marian gas – which is 98% carbon dioxide – in pained areas such as the neck, the knees and the lower back. Typically, after or during any procedure, a patient is wrapped 'like a mummy' in a number of blankets. They usually lie down during procedures, so they can rest and sometimes sleep. The doctor usually prescribes time between procedures to allow for periods of rest as well.

Most procedures are relaxing and aid in regeneration. For patient-tourists who do not suffer any 'disease' or illness, the vital relaxation and beauty are favorite programs. Otherwise, the majority of patients get relaxing mineral baths, a warming treatment, and a type of massage. A nurse told me, '99 per cent of the people balneotherapy really helps, maybe when they return home, or half a year later.'

Some patient tourists exclaimed that they felt 100% better immediately. Other couples said that they felt better within a few days.

Patient tourists

During socialism, patients or recreants were sent to Czech health spas under a doctor's orders or as a reward for good labor. The Czechs who visit Mariánské Lázně are remnants of the socialist system – they are seriously ill, usually suffering kidney disorders. The marketing director, Zusana, said, 'It is only a small number of Czechs who come to the spa with insurance with very serious illnesses, such as after an accident. Or, they pay part and the insurance pays the rest.' Since the number of Czech visitors is so small, they 'are not relevant when it comes to marketing.' Czechs who have been coming to Mariánské Lázně for years are often nostalgic for the time when the majority of patient tourists were Czech, and when nationalized insurance or unions covered each person's spa stay.

Today, most patient tourists visiting Mariánské Lázně are taking their health into their own hands, booking spa stays as they would any other vacation on the internet (Jones and Keith 2006). They are consumers concerned about their health. For instance, one German couple told me:

> We have problems with our feet and with kidney stones, and it is our first time here. We heard from a friend who was here that it was good, and so we booked a stay through the internet. We have been here for four days, and we had the gas packs, or the laughing sacks, and the mineral bath and the massage and the gymnastics. The laughing gas pack made us feel much better. We drink Caroline because the doctor told us to and we read that it was good.

As mentioned above, most Germans heard about the spa from word of mouth, travel brochures, or because it is a famous, well-known spa in Europe. Germans epitomize 'patient tourists' because they feel pain, opt for two to four week stays that include spa procedures, but they are also there to relax and enjoy excursions.

While both young and old people visit Mariánské Lázně, the majority of guests are between their 50s and their 80s. When people are older, they tend to suffer from back pain or other degenerative problems. A spa worker said, 'Your whole life you go around on your legs, and it affects your back, which is burdened. And when you have stress, you carry it in your back, the shoulders get tense and so it is all tied to the back. Every person suffers it.' The younger patient tourists who do come are described as wanting to prevent future health problems. The older patient tourists are also characterized as being more health conscious and wanting to improve themselves. Thus, guests want to generally improve themselves or rest and relax, and there are others suffering chronic pain. Martina said, 'The guests who come here are sick or they have chronic illnesses . . . there are Germans who come for prevention but the three week stays are for people with chronic diseases.' They face the usual chronic illnesses that older people tend to suffer, such as back, leg, knee, neck pain, or general rheumatism. They may also have heard that the spa specializes in kidney disorders.

Multiple Czech informants explained the huge numbers of Germans at Mariánské Lázně as due to the cheaper rates than those offered at German spas. In addition, since Germany and the Czech Republic are so close geographically, it is easy and affordable to travel to the Czech Republic. Historically speaking, it is a 'tradition' for Germans to frequent spas, especially Marienbad. Germans consider it a prestigious place to visit. A woman said, in explaining what the Germans sought out in Mariánské Lázně: 'rest, quiet, to drink the water, and to pay for the "old tradition" of Mariánské Lázně.' They seek out spa therapy in Mariánské Lázně in order to enjoy the relaxing nature of travel in another country as they benefit from cheaper spa therapies, therapies that are the same as those found in German spas.

While German spas offer the same spa procedures, Czech spas do have the special Marien gas, for which the town was named, and it is the only sort found in this region. The marketing director even said, 'Some of the Germans come only for the gas injections.' One couple said, regarding the gas injections:

> We are here for the cure, we had the massage, and gas injections, and baths. We chose Mariánské Lázně because it is very famous...We had the gas injections, and now we don't feel anything. We have problems with our knees and back and joints. We are drinking Rudolf, hopefully we will live another few years now.

The issue concerning insurance was at times unclear, since some Germans are referred to the spas by their doctors and are later reimbursed for their spa stays. However, since the majority of the German patient tourists are retired, they do not meet requirements for German spa insurance. Since the majority is self-paying, they choose to visit the cheaper Czech spas. One man said:

> I am from Dortmund, and I am retired. I used to be a banker. I have problems with my knee and shoulders and so I have mineral baths. I was here in April, and it was very good so I came back before winter starts. It helped with my problems, and I hope it will help more. I read in a book that it works for my problems, and I can't use my insurance since I don't work...Here the gas and mud are very strong and that is why it works. I get the mud on my knees and I lie down on it with my whole body. I do the gas pack, the mineral bath. I drink Rudolf and Cross for my digestion.

Since this man is paying out of pocket, he, like many other retired Germans, chose to combine a more affordable spa therapy with vacation.

Since the treatments are more affordable for people paying out of their own pockets, Germans are acting as consumers vacationing and receiving health treatments. Some couples say they come to Mariánské Lázně because it treats a wider variety of illnesses, and has better tasting mineral waters. One German couple said, 'The procedures are completely the same in Germany, and we like it here since nearly all the sicknesses are included in the package.' Others said they came to Mariánské Lázně because it is so beautiful. However, the main issue is that German spas cannot compete with Czech prices, while Czech spas can compete with the quality of German spas.

The patient tourists who visit Mariánské Lázně are spoken of as very satisfied customers, since they return repeatedly for treatment – sometimes as frequently as once every six months, as the informant cited above, but usually every year or every other year. The majority of the patient tourists come for spa treatment, and when they are inside the hotels they are often seen sporting their robes. Outside, on the colonnade and in the parks, they usually carry their souvenir cups for their drinking cures.

Packaging balneotherapy

Indications and contraindications at Mariánské Lázně have increased since the privatization of Czech spas. Thus, while the balneotherapy procedures have remained constant, the indication list of Mariánské Lázně reflects the expansion of spa industries into the realm of tourism. The key is to market spas to a larger number of people. In 1992 and 1998, new indications of gynecology and post-operation rehabilitation were added, due to the efforts made by one head doctor. But some doctors would rather limit Mariánské Lázně's indications to only kidney problems and back pain. These doctors are resisting the popularization of balneotherapy for the sake of tourism since they fear demedicalizing spa therapies completely.

Doctors and health workers were reluctant to say that balneotherapy as a healing regime has changed. However, it is apparent that the role of the doctor is changing. Some doctors were even leaning toward the marketing side of spa business – they wanted to open a balneological spa in Las Vegas. Doctors are faced with a new group of leaders in the spas: spa hotel managers and marketing corporations who are reformulating the spa industry. More popular than medical courses in balneotherapy are the managerial courses in balneology at the master's level of university education.

Since there are more managerial programs and balneotherapy is the basis of a tourism industry, the financing of balneotherapy has decidedly changed. It is now big business. Doctors talked about this as having a detrimental effect on spa medicine. Now, marketing directors and advertising executives are creating new spa packages for tourists that do not take into consideration indications or contraindications for certain procedures. Treatment specialists often shook their heads when they found a patient with varicose veins lying on their massage table.

Spa hotels now offer 'packages' that have 20 procedures for a two-week stay, and they are already priced for the guests. While physicians recommend three to four weeks for an effective treatment, guests can now choose from a range of one to two week programs such as 'relaxation' or 'beauty week' or 'anti-stress'. The anti-stress package, 'a week of natural spa treatment for high demand persons,' and a vital spa stay for ladies are both newly developed by Zusana and her marketing team. However, doctors claim that if you only visit the spa for one week, you will feel worse.

Beauty is one of the new emphases of spa packages. Beauty treatments include wraps, or natural sources that can be used to treat skin problems like eczema. Minerals themselves are said to be beautifying. Beauty salons can be found inside each hotel and spa, and laser surgery is even offered at two of the spa hotels. While beauty treatments are not listed among balneotherapy procedures, spas are trying to highlight these programs for new kinds of guests. Spa packages are moving away from purely medical indications such as kidney disorders to appeal to a younger, non-German clientele.

Now, tourists can purchase packages that promise them an overall 'health, wellness, medicine, beauty and fitness' regimen. In addition to beauty, the vacations at Mariánské Lázně emphasize active relaxation and leisure – which are, again, non-medical and general. One can see a palpable change from a public health system to a health tourism industry. As a necessary part of this structural change, one detects subtle shifts and consequent incongruities as doctors struggle for control over the medical portion of spa hotels. As marketing groups create new packages for a general clientele, balneotherapy is no longer in the sole purview of medicine.

Disbelieving tourists

Related to the issue of the doctor's authority in the spa, the changes occurring with the privatization of tourism entails the entrance of 'tourists' to Mariánské Lázně, who are not seeking spa treatment but who are still staying at spa hotels. A very different group of new tourists in Mariánské Lázně are British and American guests. Though both British and Americans enjoyed spas in the nineteenth century, the spa tradition faded in both countries. The marketing manager said, 'The Germans know what to do here at the spa, they know the routine. But the English don't really and so it is different and harder, we need to learn their needs.' Indeed, in British travel brochures, the spas are marketed as a second part of a two city Czech tour, and Mariánské Lázně is described as having natural walking paths. The spa portion of the facilities is never emphasized in these brochures. The marketing director also stated, 'I wanted to cut out the gas injections in brochures for the English clients, because it makes the spa look like a hospital and they won't want to come. The doctors understood that the Germans love the injections, but that the English don't. Indeed, British guests mentioned this at welcome meetings, 'the gas injections sound horrible' they would gasp, as they flipped through hotel pamphlets.

A British travel agency representative, Iasen (pronounced Ya-sen), was instructed the year before British tourists started arriving in Mariánské Lázně to take pictures of only the scenery without any buildings in them, to emphasize the 'natural' beauty of the town. A British guest said, 'We enjoy coming to spas not because of the treatments but because of the culture.' Although British guests are offered complimentary massages, most British men decline.

Most British guests, like the Germans, were older and retired, often traveling as couples. However, as a new group of patient tourists, they faced several barriers. Mainly, for them as well as for Saudis and Arabs, not enough people spoke English for them in the hotels and the shops. While some British guests found this to be an entertaining challenge, others complained that they were bored and had no one with whom to talk. One man at a hotel who was on vacation, but also had a bit of neck pain, exclaimed that the anthropologist was only the second person he had met who speaks English. One British woman who was actually visiting her mother said there should be more people who speak English, because her husband was lonely.

In addition to the language barrier, the spa hotels proved too strict, formal and unrelenting to the more casual British holiday guests. For example, it is customary for guests to visit the doctor their first day upon arrival to the spa. However, since the British guests were not there for spa treatments, they would feel alarmed after being sent up to have their blood pressure taken. The British travel agency representative Iasen said, 'The people are here for a holiday and it took me an entire summer to tell each reception person that they are *not* to send my guests directly to the nurse to have their blood pressure taken. They are here for a holiday and they don't need the stress of the blood pressure test.' He finally had to tell the guests at the airport directly to ignore the receptionists' instructions.

The menu offerings were equally strict. Iasen confided, 'I have complaints from guests about the food as well, they are not flexible. Here, they have dinner only from five thirty to seven thirty and the people don't want to eat that early on their holiday, especially if it doesn't get dark until ten. They are inflexible about the choices as well, having a cold plate for dinner. I have to tell the hotels that these people are not on diets, they are on holiday and they want to eat.' There were certain nights when only fruit and cheese were served, and the British guests felt guilty when they sat eating normal, large meals in front of the spa dieters.

Similar to the 'catastrophe' that was the disconnect between British guests' needs and the spa services, there was a problem with different notions of 'spa'. The kinds of procedures that are offered in Mariánské Lázně differ radically from the types of treatments and relaxing procedures offered in American 'spas'. In American spas, relaxing hour-long hot stone therapy massages with aromatherapy, or other pampering elements, are the main component.

For instance, one afternoon in New Spa, a New York forty-something career woman was extremely distraught with one spa hotel where participant observation was being conducted. She ranted and raved about how inflexible the spa was. She had traveled to Mariánské Lázně through a New York travel agency, had booked a week-long 'spa' stay in *Nové Lázně* (New Spa), and found it to be incomprehensible. She complained to the nurse, 'I paid two thousand dollars for this!' She was upset because she had bought her trip in New York, where they have a travel agency that specializes in travel to Eastern European spas. She had been told that she could get help with her back with the peat pack, but upon arrival the Czech doctor diagnosed gymnastics. Group aerobic exercises contrasted sharply with her image of relaxing mud baths. She said, exasperated, 'I paid for certain procedures and I didn't get them. I have had arguments with people since I got here yesterday. They won't take the voucher that said I paid already, they want me to pay again.' In the spa hotel's brochure, hour-long massages as well as mud baths are listed as possible procedures. However, due to the actual expense of using so much mud, the hotels never actually give complete mud baths. Also, this New Yorker was given a partial massage and a mineral bath, procedures she found unnecessary. As her rant drew to a close, she finished by saying, 'I have a tub in New York, I don't need a bath.' Again, an American does not expect a room temperature, stinky mineral bath to be part of a spa package.

It is obvious from this woman's experience the disjuncture that exists between the spas in the Czech Republic and those in America, and the problems that occur when an American purchases a spa package. The procedures differ dramatically, although the prices for the Czech spas are much less expensive. Indeed, a doctor said in an interview, 'In Central Europe is the largest tradition here of spas. It is a catastrophe when people come from England or America and expect something else.'

Commodified health care

There is a general consensus among spa doctors and employees that balneotherapy has become commodified. During socialism, medicine was available to all workers. Now, it only matters who can afford these increasingly expensive treatments. The key for marketers of Czech spas is to market spas to a larger number of people. In this process, spas are demedicalized. Some doctors are resisting this popularization of balneotherapy for the sake of tourism. Thus, while balneotherapy entails the same therapeutic elements, the commercial context in which it exists has shaped a new kind of health tourism. Now, treatments can include traditional forms of balneotherapy, but also acupuncture, massage therapy, plastic surgery, herbal medicines and fitness training. One doctor said, 'Today, balneotherapy is more or less a business with more and more procedures, we are no longer specialized.'

Now that spas are privatized, the patients are consumers who return nearly annually because they are satisfied with the spa services. Before, Czech patients or recreants visited spas under their insurance, thus they were forced to follow doctor's orders. A German patient tourist said, 'before, the difference was that you had to see a doctor before getting the cure, whereas now you can pay for what you want.' Now the German patient tourists who come are referred to as the ones who 'know how to pay.' With the loss of universal health insurance coverage of spas and the increase in cost, Czechs are a minority of patient tourists at the spas. Some people argue that spas are improved, because anyone can come, whereas before you needed a prescription. More often, however, it is the patient tourist, not 'anyone,' who can afford to visit. At the end of the fieldwork, the anthropologist went to the doctor's office to set up her own spa stay. He turned to her as she walked into his office and simply asked, 'Do you have money?' It is apparent, now, that what is important is not necessarily the health status of the patient tourist, but rather, his or her financial status.

Since the end of socialism, various scholars have written about the elasticity of memory and the various ways in which nostalgia, or 'ostalgia', for socialism has surfaced in Central Europe (Hahn 2002; Berdahl 1999; Gal and Kligman 2000). Berdahl (1999) has considered nostalgia to be a discourse of resistance. As Gal and Kligman (2000, 87) noted, people in Central Europe have 'nostalgia for the material security . . . and the relative egalitarianism that the communist system fostered'. In the case of Mariánské Lázně, nostalgia for full insurance coverage for spa stays and for the presence of more Czech patient tourists in the town were the main themes.

Since Czech spas are traditionally 'medical' in nature, they must shift their focus toward the global trends of spas to compete in the global market. Czech spas must offer more generalized relaxing and anti-stress packages of therapies. The commercialization of spas, however, marginalizes the spa doctor, as the marketing groups try to draw different clienteles to the spa towns. The trend is away from kidney diseases toward youth and beauty and anti-stress programs. In this way, the spas can appeal to even more people who are not necessarily 'sick'. Medical tourism is diversifying in a privatized spa industry where chronically ill patients are being treated in addition to vacation seekers. People seeking health care, relaxation or preventative care find affordable health care and vacations at this one locale in Central Europe.

This trend is a continuation, and not a break, from the socialist trend of allowing recreants to come and enjoy spa therapies in town. However, the majority of the doctors anticipated spa medicine becoming even 'more commercial.' One doctor bemoaned the fact that it has 'changed for the worse, because before it was for treating and now it is more for profit . . . During communism it was about care for the person.' This nostalgia reveals the tensions that arise within a changing field of spa medicine as it is being popularized and commercialized within a post-socialist health tourism context.

Acknowledgements

This paper is based on the anthropologist's dissertation research that was conducted during the summers of 2000, 2001, and all of 2002. The research was partially funded by a Fellowship for Language and Area Studies. The research was approved by the University of Pittsburgh's Institutional Review Board.

Thanks are due to all informants from Mariánské Lázně, and especially landlords who still provided a home for the anthropologist during her too infrequent visits. Informants will not be named in order to protect their privacy. However, many residents, doctors, nurses, spa workers, and patients took the time to talk to about their understandings of balneotherapy.

Thanks are also due to Dr Joseph Alter, who proved to be the best graduate school advisor. His thoughtful support continues to this day. Other valuable professors from the University of Pittsburgh include Dr Nicole Constable, Dr Robert Hayden, and Dr Andrew Strathern. The anthropologist's close-knit cohort, especially Frayda Cohen, Leah Voors, Sarah Thurston, and Angela Lockard Reed, and their friendship were invaluable. Finally, the anthropologist would not have been able to complete her work without the emotional and material support of her husband, Eric Wiltrout.

Conflict of interest: none.

Note

1. There has been considerable debate regarding the proper term for medical tourism. Some have argued that tourism connotes frivolous leisure without recognizing the serious medical issues some travelers have (Matorras 2005; Inhorn and Birenbaum-Carmeli 2008). This debate hinges on older debates regarding a distinction between tourists and travelers (Urry 2002; Errington and Gewertz 2004; Gmelch 2004). However, some have claimed that medical tourism does entail aspects of tourism (Connell 2006; Pennings 2005). For the purposes of this paper, the term used will be health tourism, since spa treatments are non-invasive and some tourists only go to spa towns to relax, thus preventing future health problems.

References

Aron, Cindy S. 1999. *Working at play: A history of vacations in the United States*. New York: Oxford University Press.

Berdahl, Daphne. 1999. *Where the world ended: Re-unification and identity in the German borderland*. Berkeley: University of California Press.

Carter, Frank W. 1991. Czechoslovakia. In *Tourism and economic development in Eastern Europe and the Soviet Union*, ed. D. Hall, London: Belhaven Press.

Connell, John. 2006. Medical tourism: sea, sun, sand and . . . surgery. *Tourism Management* 27: 1093–100.

Errington, Frederick, and Deborah Gewertz. 2004. Tourism and anthropology in a postmodern world. In *Tourists and tourism: A reader*, ed. Sharon Bohn Gmelch. Long Grove: Waveland Press.

Gal, Susan, and Gail Kligman. 2000. *The politics of gender after socialism*. Princeton: Princeton University Press.

Gmelch, Sharon Bohn. 2004. Why tourism matters. In *Tourists and tourism: A reader*, ed. Sharon Bohn Gmelch, Long Grove: Waveland Press.

Hahn, Chris, ed. 2002. *Postsocialism: Ideals, ideologies and practices in Eurasia*. New York: Routledge.

Inhorn, Marcia C., and Daphna Birenbaum-Carmeli. 2008. Assisted reproductive technologies and culture change. *Annual Review of Anthropology* 37: 177–96.

Jirásek, Karel. 1979. *Ceskoslovenské Lázne*. Praha: Olympia.

Jones, C.A., and L.G. Keith. 2006. Medical tourism and reproductive outsourcing: The dawning of a new paradigm for health care. *International Journal of Fertility and Women's Medicine* 51, no. 6: 251–5.

Matorras, Roberto. 2005. Reproductive exile versus reproductive tourism. *Human Reproduction* 20, no. 12: 3571.

Nepustil, Bohumír. 1949 *Czechoslovak public health services*, compiled from data supplied by the Ministry of Health.

Noack, Christian. 2006. Coping with the tourist: Planned and 'wild' mass tourism on the Soviet Black Sea coast. In *Turizm: The Russian and East European tourist under capitalism and socialism*, ed. A.E. Gorsuch and D.P. Koeneker, Ithaca: Cornell University Press.

Pennings, Guido. 2005. Reply to 'Reproductive exile versus reproductive tourism'. *Human Reproduction* 20, no. 12: 3571–2.

Prerovský, K. 1957. *Czechoslovak spas*. Pragne: Mír 1.

Urry, John. 2002. *The tourist gaze*. 2nd edn. London: Sage Publications.

Of relics, body parts and laser beams: the German Heilpraktiker and his Ayurvedic spa

Harish Naraindas

*Centre for the Study of Social Systems, School of Social Sciences,
Jawaharlal Nehru University, New Delhi, India*

This paper examines the twin German institutions of the Kur (spa), and the 'lay' licensed healing practitioner or Heilpraktiker. Through an ethnography of a Heilpraktiker and his Ayurvedic spa in a small catholic village in Germany, where patients arrive in person or as body parts by post, it examines the poly-therapeutics of the practitioner, who seems to combine in his being a dizzy array of diagnostic and therapeutic possibilities. It argues that the while the Ayurvedic spa can be seen as a kind of variation of the traditional German Kur, the Heilpraktiker's poly-therapy has to draw upon the special nature of the practice of medicine in Germany, symbolised in part by the very figure of the Heilpraktiker. It attempts to show that the practitioner's panoply of therapies is partly a symptom of an epistemic impasse at the heart of biomedicine, leading patients on an itinerant quest toward different therapeutic locales, such as the Kur, or to different therapeutic possibilities, such as the ones offered by the Heilpraktiker. But while the Kur and the Heilpraktiker would be either fringe or alternative in the Anglo-American world, in Germany the Kur is part of orthodox medicine, and the Heilpraktiker is a legal entity; and the two together redraw and make fuzzy what elsewhere seem to be clearly drawn boundaries between medicine and the spa, between pleasure and therapy, and medicine and alternative medicine.

In the centre of a catholic village of around 800 households in northern Germany is a small roadside shrine of the Virgin with the Infant. Behind it stands a building with a bright red roof, through the centre of which rises a 'Hindu temple tower'. It houses a German Heilpraktiker (healing practitioner) and his spa. One enters an enclosed courtyard through a curtain of multicoloured glass beads to be greeted by soft music, with Ayurvedic treatment wings for men and women on either side. Beyond it is a foyer that functions during the day as a waiting room and in the evening as a lecture room where resident patients are educated in either a particular facet of the Ayurvedic treatment, or offered an explanation of one of the many diagnostic and therapeutic procedures that the practitioner carries out in tandem with the Ayurvedic ones.

Towards the close of a scheduled two-hour interview with the Heilpraktiker in the foyer, a female patient walks in and is witness to the interview. The interview on his practice doubles up as an unstated introduction to the waiting patient and thus allows the author easy access into the consulting room. The patient walks in and sits on a stool beside a large desk with a laptop. The laptop is attached to a headphone and to what looks like an external hard drive on which it says 'ITA scan'.[1] These devices in turn are attached through a series of wires to two small contraptions: a small metal canister and a second small cylindrical metal device that, according to the Heilpraktiker, emits a laser beam. The Heilpraktiker wraps the headphones around the patient's ears, thus completing a loop between the laptop, the ITA scan external drive, the canister, and the laser beam. He then proceeds to diagnose the patient. The diagnosis appears as a series of colourful scans on the computer screen of first simulated body parts – heart, brain, kidney, lung, liver, etc – and then of systems – endocrine, vascular, etc. The condition of each organ and system is colour-coded, ranging from yellow – healthy – to black – unhealthy. Having thus diagnosed the patient, the programme then proceeds to simulate a therapy. The simulated therapy is then beamed through the laser to the canister into which the practitioner has placed homeopathic sugar pills in a transparent plastic pouch. The pouch of these irradiated pills is then removed from the canister, is necked with a rubber band, and handed over to the patient. The whole process takes about 20 to 30 minutes.

This spa was part of an initial survey chosen as an example of a Heilpraktiker running an Ayurvedic spa in Germany. Having driven a great distance to interview him about his Ayurvedic practice, which was indeed the fulcrum around which his spa was built, the Heilpraktiker's consulting room came as a surprise. The fortuitous presence of the patient, and an impromptu plea to witness a consultation, followed by her consent, led to a consulting room that was an inventive panoply of gadgets, Gurus, Virgins and other paraphernalia: a virtual therapeutic armoury that the Heilpraktiker deployed to help his patients with their distress. It was this panoply[2] that led the author to visit and stay at the spa next summer, to wrestle with the question of what the panoply meant for both practitioner and patients, how it functioned in an Ayurvedic spa, and what place it occupied in the German therapeutic landscape.

Hence, this essay will revolve around two poles: the Ayurvedic spa in Germany as a particular kind of therapeutic locale that is seemingly far removed from the traditional spa built around water, and the poly-therapeutics of the practitioner who seems to combine in his being a dizzy array of diagnostic and therapeutic possibilities, producing in the bargain a mangled medical episteme that needs to be addressed. The argument, in advance, is that the Ayurvedic spa can be seen as a kind of variation of the traditional German Kur (spa), built initially and historically around the 'taking of waters' and situated around a Bad (mineral bath). The other diagnostic and therapeutic procedures of the Heilpraktiker, which will form the other pole of this essay, will have to draw upon the peculiar nature of the practice of medicine in Germany, symbolised in part by the figure of the Heilpraktiker as a legal entity who comes into being in 1939 (Unschuld 1980). This local register, while cardinal, incorporates the global register of the practice of medicine worldwide in so far as the poly-therapeutics of the Heilpraktiker may be seen as a symptom of the conundrum in which an idealised picture of the practice of Schulmedizin (school medicine)[3] is caught, leading patients on an itinerant quest toward alternative therapies, and practitioners to offer a rich palette, or panoply, of therapies in an attempt to address what orthodox biomedicine seems both unable and unwilling to address. Toward the end of this essay, this conundrum will not only be made apparent, but the reader will see what bearing it has on patients' itinerant quests, and how the German Heilpraktiker is both a singular and a general symptom of both a malaise and a cure. The essay will begin, however, by attempting to situate the spa as part of general therapeutic practice and then see how the German spa or Kur may be located in this landscape before addressing the Ayurvedic spa in Germany. The essay will return at the end to the Heilpraktiker and his panoply, and attempt to show that they are part homologues of the German Kur; and that both the Kur and the Heilpraktiker should be seen as part of a larger German therapeutic landscape if one is to make sense of them.

Of medicine and wellness: situating the spa in the practice of medicine

In the continental European context, as opposed to the Anglo-American context, the neat distinction between biomedicine and alternative medicine, or between medicine and wellness, becomes fuzzy, especially with respect to 'spa medicine'. An idealised picture of biomedicine, which may safely be said to be the practice of post war Anglo-American medicine writ large, is made fuzzy by the fact that spa therapy is itself part of orthodox medical practice in large parts of Europe (Maretzki 1987; Weisz 2001). The contrast between these two worlds is best captured by the fact that there are nearly 300 Bad towns in Germany (Thornton and Brutscher 2009) with 273,000 annual visits, and 50% of these visits are reimbursed by insurance (Weisz 2001). The German Kur system, in other words, is the third leg of the German National Health System, with the other two being the *Hausarzt* or house doctor (GP), and the hospital system. In the last 40 years about nine million Germans have supposedly benefited from its presence (Weisz 2001) and, according to the European Spa Association, the German Kurorte and thermal baths currently employ 350,000 people and account for 30% of overnight stays in terms of tourism in Germany.

Italy is next in terms of spa goers with 180,000 annual visits, with two thirds of these being reimbursed; and France is third with about 64,000 visits, with 90% of these French visits being reimbursed 'by the national insurance system' (Weisz 2001). This, as Weisz points out in the French case, is partly made possible by the fact that the spa is 'medicalised' and becomes part of the practice of medicine in France (Weisz 2001). Hence, in large parts of Europe, unlike the rest of the world, spa going is not merely an old practice but a current one and is paid for by either the State or insurance. This is increasingly under threat, leading to its current transformation, which can be loosely described as a movement from 'medicine' to 'wellness'.

A telling example of this contrast between the European and Anglo-American model of medicine is provided by the Czech spa that Speier (2011) describes, where the new breed of British and American 'vacationers' in Marienbad are shown to be rather confused when they arrive, mainly because they have no experience of the European Kur and hence of 'spa etiquette'. This is not surprising, as in 1992 only 5500 persons in Britain used the spa as a cure and none were paid for by National Health Service (Weisz 2001, 452). Speier goes on to record how the recent presence of the British and Americans in the Czech spa, who may be called 'vacationer-patients' (and many are not 'patients' at all) rather than the European 'patient-vacationers', leads to a litany of lament from the spa doctors about the demise of the spa as serious medical therapy. This litany, which marks a transition in the nature of the Czech spa, may be easily generalised as being symptomatic of the transformation of the spa in Europe.

While it is moot as to whether this transition and transformation will ever be fully effected in Europe, given its long history of spa going, the effect of this transformation can be clearly seen in the attempted rechristening of the German Kur. From January 2000, the word Kur is no longer officially part of the recognised lexicon for social insurance. The new term, or rather terms, are Reha (rehabilitation), which invokes a period of recovery from clearly perceived organic pathology (a stroke, for example) on the one side, a side that is increasingly carved out and defended by doctors as serious medical therapy in opposition to the Kur,[4] and the words Prevention and Wellness on the other side, where prevention appears as the medical side of the pole, while Wellness is the recreational side. The latter two, called Prävention im Kurort and Wellness im Kurort are the quality control stamps given by the Deutschen Heilbäderverbandes or the Deutschen Tourismusverbandes (Deutscher-heilbaederverband, or the German Therapeutic Baths Association 2010).

Having said that, it appears that Kurorte (Kur places) and Badärzte (Bad doctors) are still a recognised category in so far as patients may still go directly to a Badarzt and have therapies prescribed, which may be paid for by insurance along with no more than €13 per day for board and lodge (€21 for a child): a far cry from the case in the 1980s when Germans had a virtual right to a fully paid Kur every few years. While the well-recognized exception to this seems to the 'Mother and Child Kur', (although the official terminology is 'Mother/Father/Child medical prevention and rehabilitation'), the German Therapeutic Baths Association (Deutscher-heilbaederverband 2010) presents the following typology: at one end is the Mother and Child rehabilitation that seems to be processed through the pension fund. At the other end is a rehabilitation that is arranged directly by the hospital, for example in instances following a stroke or a surgery, which may be paid either by the health insurance or the pension fund. In between these two extremes is that grey area between inpatient and outpatient centres where the Kurorte and the rehabilitation centres compete and distinguish themselves from each other, leading to a new set of hybrids like Reha-Kur and Wellness-Kur. In any case, in the case of both these institutions, the first port of call is either a doctor (a Hausartzt and usually a Facharzt (specialist)), followed by a wrestling with the health insurance and the pension fund to determine the possibility, and the length and the place of the Kur, although the normal length is for three weeks.

This shrinking of the 'official' Kur system has not meant that the spa industry as a whole has declined or indeed that it is declining. On the contrary, it is growing by leaps and bounds, as is clear from the figures put out by the International Spa Association (ISPA). These figures indicate that the number of spas in the US actually grew at an annual rate of 21% from 1995–1999 and continues to show strong growth. Aggregate industry revenues grew by 114% between 1999 and 2001. The size of the United States spa industry in 2001 was estimated at 9632 locations; in 2000, that number was only 5689. In 2002, there was a grand re-opening of Bath in England. But this phenomenal growth in the US and the re-launching of Bath in the UK would typically not be seen as being part of 'medicine' for two interconnected reasons: spa visits may not be supported by either insurance or the NHS; and its therapeutic arsenal rather than being 'confined' to the 'science of balneology' would now include a host of seemingly exotic possibilities. Both these would place it under alternative therapy or wellness tourism. This is evident from the fact that in the UK, although 60 patients travelled abroad to the Avene Dermatological spa in 2004 (one can apply to the NHS through form E11 or E12) for chronic eczema, only two were funded by the NHS.

Methodological and historiographical implications of the spa

The contemporary difference between the European and Anglo-American world of spas also has methodological implications. What the study of the contemporary European spa shows is that the demise of the spa, or rather its exit from the world of medicine in the Anglo-American world, leads to a normative construction of the spa as part of alternative therapy at best, or part of the wellness industry at worst. Since this is how the spa is seen (and in fact has supposedly come to be) in this world, it leads Anglo-American scholarship, or scholars with this (post-war) Anglo-American model as the tacit frame of reference, to 'explain' its persistence in Europe. These explanations have proved rather useful, however, especially the one by George Weisz, who, as pointed out earlier, argues that it is the 'medicalisation' of the spa in France, enabled partly by the strength of the spa industry, that leads to its incorporation or continuation in orthodox medical practice, albeit a fringe one. If, however, the European practice of medicine and especially the German practice of medicine is made the norm, then spa practice, which was part of medical practice in nineteenth century Europe (Mackaman 1998), and continued to be so until very recently, is de-medicalised in the Anglo-American world, then it is this that needs to be explained.

One of the consequences of this de-medicalisation may well be the appearance of health 'tourism' and 'wellness' as an 'alternative' industry. In other words, what was once orthodox medical practice is 'squeezed out' and re-appears as heterodox medical practice, especially in the Anglo-American world. This argument may then be extended to cover a gamut of what are now called alternative medical practices but particularly so for climate, travel and locale as therapy, all of which appear as legitimate medical theory and practice as late as the late nineteenth and early twentieth century, and all of which are cardinal to the contemporary German Kur system, which encompasses much more than the use of mineral water for either bathing or consumption.

The discourse on climate is a good example of how, in the nineteenth century, climate was central as a mode of reasoning both in the causation of disease and its cure (Naraindas 1996). This preoccupation with climate rested not merely on scenic therapeutic locales, or merely in terms of good and clean air, but in terms of its direct bearing on epidemics and fevers on the one hand and on the body's physiological functions on the other (Naraindas 1996). The latter, particularly under the twin nineteenth-century figures of the consumptive and the invalid, occupied itself with providing a casual scheme and a therapeutic format under the notion of 'change of air'. The following works are suggestive of the range: James Clark's (1830) *The influence of climate in the prevention and cure of chronic diseases, more particularly of the chest and digestive organs*; James Johnson's (1831) *Change of air, or the philosophy of traveling*; John Thorowgood's (1868) *The climatic treatment of consumption and chronic lung diseases*; and Weber and Foster's (1896) *Climate in the treatment of disease*. The nineteenth-century spa has to be seen as belonging to this larger landscape of what may be called medical geography or geographical pathology (Boudin 1856; Davidson 1892), where mineral waters, the air, temperature and locale all fused to produce a vast therapeutic landscape differentiated according to diseases. The sanatorium is but one example of this therapeutic landscape with the others being the hill station in the tropics, the voyage and the furlough from the tropics, and the grand tour in Europe (Naraindas 1996).[5] The tropics were the extreme version of climate and locale impinging on health, creating in the bargain a moral meteorology, the most well-known fallout of which was the anxiety over acclimatisation[6] and the possibility of tropical colonisation. But the preoccupation with climate was equally true in Europe and was part of a more general carving up of space into the pathological and the healthy (Naraindas 1996).

Vincent Priessnitz, and his 'rediscovery' in Silesia in 1831 of cold common water as a cure and eventually as a therapeutic format, which was initially called the cold water cure and later christened as hydrotherapy, presents another genealogy of plain cold water (as opposed to 'hot' mineral water) as a spa cure, which included the natural elements air and earth. This is elaborated by Father Sebastian Kneipp and many other Germans, and in fact this branch is now the Kneipp therapy that Germans use as a home remedy. Here again, it would be a grave mistake to see common cold water as only addressing what may be called the chronic conditions of the palsies and the rheumatisms (as the titles above with respect to climate may suggest). The complex genealogy of cold water as cure (both through bathing and drinking in its late modern form), usually traced to John Floyer's work (*psykhroloysia*) of 1702, finds one of its clearest statement in Tobias Smollet, who in 1752 argued for its mechanical rather than its mineral properties as being responsible for effecting a cure (Cayleff 1987). While this did not mark the demise of its mineral philosophy as is evident by its transmutation and appropriation by chemists from the late eighteenth century (Hamlin 1990), what it introduces is another strand and in fact a whole social movement built around common water that Cayleff records for nineteenth-century America. But here again, historiography, based on contemporary concerns and presumptions, is selective in so far as it does not address the fact that common water was used as therapy for smallpox and generally for fever in the eighteenth century (Hancocke 1722). It is difficult to say whether this is due to the introduction of smallpox inoculation into England first from Turkey in the 1710s and then from India where it comes accompanied by the water cure (Holwell 1767; Naraindas 2003), or whether these provide a further fillip to a pre-existing practice. But what is clear is that the 'acme' of the water cure movement is the smallpox epidemic of Gloucester in 1893, where hydrotherapy pits itself against vaccination in a general climate of protest against vaccination, orchestrated throughout the length and breath of England by the anti-vaccination leagues.[7]

Hence, many of the ingredients and therapeutic formats of what is now called spa therapy, but especially climate, locale and water in its mineral and common form – 'revived' in the eighteenth century under the sign of the Hippocratic triad of 'airs, waters and places' – are evident today in the current classification of the German Kur system into the five broad rubrics of Mineral und Moorheilbäder (Mineral and Mud baths),[8] Heilklimatische Kuorte (Healing Climates), Seeheil- und Seebäder

(Sea cures and Sea baths), and Kneippheilbäder and Kneipkuorte (Kneipp Kur places) and Luftkuorte (Aerotherapy Kurs).

The French and German cases are particularly interesting, since the thesis is that the spa 'survives' in France, where it becomes the science of balneology, due its medicalisation (Weisz 2001). But Weisz is quite aware that unlike the fully medicalised spa in France 'the German spa seems to be a curious admixture of mainstream medical activity and alternative medical practice aimed at health tourism and wellness' (Weisz 2001, 452).[9] While this may well be the case, and instructive in so far as the words 'alternative', 'wellness' and 'tourism' are expectedly clubbed together in Weisz, it is necessary in the German case to widen the ambit – both conceptually and legally – of what constitutes 'mainstream medicine'. This might result in seeing this 'curious admixture' not only in the German spa but also in the practice of German medicine in general. This in turn may have an important bearing on conceptualising the boundary between 'medicine' on the one hand and 'alternative' 'wellness' and 'tourism' on the other, and generally between 'medicine' and 'alternative medicine', and finally between the university trained Schulmedizin doctor and the German Heilpraktiker.

The fuzzy boundaries between orthodox and heterodox medical practices in Germany

Having thus signalled that the practice of orthodox medicine in large parts of Europe includes spa therapy, in the German case it also appears to include a number of other therapies that in the Anglo-American world would be labelled 'alternative'. In three articles written in the 1980s, Thomas Maretzki (1987, 1989; Maretzki and Seidler 1985) demonstrates that the German practice of medicine, as opposed to its American variant, includes not only the Kur but also various naturopathic therapies, including homeopathy, Kneipp therapy and many others. Maretzki says that 'in the United States "alternative medicine" is mainly found outside of both academic medicine and professional practice; in West Germany, however, it survives as part of professional practice, although it is neither acknowledged nor condoned by academic medicine (Schulmedizin), which sets the ideal, though ever-changing standards of the profession' (Maretzki 1989, 22). This world of academic medicine and professional practice, as pointed out earlier, is broadly divided into the three categories of the Hausarzt (GP), 'who usually has no hospital privileges' (Maretzki 1989, 22), the university/hospital doctor, and the Bad/Kur doctor (Badearzt), to which should be added the Facharzt (specialist in private practice). While the Kur/Bad doctor may be seen as being lower down the hierarchy in terms of prestige, the fact remains that it is a medical specialisation.

While the Kur is part of the university curriculum, doctors can also acquire competence, through a process of training and certification outside the University, in a number of other therapies or 'therapeutic systems' such as acupuncture, homeopathy, Kineseology, Kirlian photography, Naturheilkunde (nature healing or naturopathy) and increasingly Ayurveda, that they then combine with Schulmedizin therapies as part of their practice. Maretzki's claim, confirmed by extensive personal observation, means that one is unlikely to meet a German doctor who only practices Schulmedizin in its idealised Anglophone variant!

These Schulmedizin poly-therapists are under an umbrella organisation called the Hufeland Society (Hufeland-Gesellscahft). This society initially came up with a list of complementary therapies in the form of a book called the Hufeland-Leistungsverzeichnis der Besonderen Therapierichtungen (HLÄ). While this was initially meant to assist doctors to write bills for privately insured patients, it has become over time a quasi-legal reference book for insurance companies and thus allows patients who pay out of pocket to seek a reimbursement from the insurance companies. While the HLA and its reimbursement schedule is not 'good in law', it is good in convention and more or less sacrosanct as far as the insurance companies are concerned. The HLA in turn is modelled on what Maretzki (1989) calls the *Gebührenordnung für Ärzte* (or GOÄ, which can be translated as Schedule of Tariffs for Physicians) that functions as a prototype and first reference for the Schulmedizin doctors, with the other one being the official nosology or the International Classification of Diseases (ICD). A doctor practising medicine in Germany is by law allowed to bill for his medical services only according to the GOÄ. In practice, a doctor's bill according to this GOÄ is only written for privately insured patients; in the case of statutory health-insurance the remuneration for doctors' services is negotiated differently between the health-insurances and the Association of Statutory Health Insurance Physicians (this expression is given in the dictionary for *Kassenärztliche Vereinigung*). Between these two books, the HLÄ and GOÄ, the German health care system attempts to cover the population as broadly as possible through a combination of statutory health insurance and private health insurance, which is very different from the NHS.

In other words, if the Kur functions within the ambit of orthodox medical practice, these 'alternative therapies', or in the German case 'medical specialities' learnt outside the official university Schulmedizin curriculum, also function within orthodox medicine and like the Kur are regulated, monitored and reimbursed by insurance, although not to the same degree or as easily.[10] In the case of 'conventional therapies', the patient never gets to see the bill as it is paid by the statutory health insurance, unless the patient is privately insured; while in the latter case he often, if not invariably, pays out of pocket and is then reimbursed, though not always or not necessarily fully.

The licensed lay practitioner or the German Heilpraktiker

But Schulmedizin with its various curricular and 'extra-curricular' medical specialities does not exhaust the medically reimbursable German therapeutic landscape. In order to capture the distinctive nature of German medical practice one must also include the lay person, who with a minimum of nine years of formal schooling (the Hauptschulabschluss),[11] is allowed to practice medicine, provided he is able to pass an exam and then a viva voce administered by the State. Brought into being in 1939 (Unschuld 1980), this non-university, lay, licensed healer, called the Heilpraktiker, is – as Maretzki (1989) puts it – a 'parallel therapeutic resource' and a 'trained and licensed lay practitioner'. While Maretzki does not indicate how and where he is trained, it is clear that what he is trained in is often no different from the extra-curricular competences that the Schulmedizin doctor acquires as their 'diagnostic and therapeutic services overlap with those of physicians trained in naturopathic and homeopathic medicine' (Maretzki 1989). In other words, it transpires that in Germany there is a 'licensed' lay practitioner who practises what are called alternative practices in the Anglophone world, and these alternative practices are also practised by university trained doctors who acquire them as extra-curricular medical specialities, thus offering German patients a 'plurality of therapeutic modalities...*all paid for* by government and private health insurance' (Maretzki 1989, emphasis added).

If this were to be represented diagrammatically, it would appear as a Venn diagram of two intersecting circles called Schulmedizin doctors and Heilpraktikers, with the common area being their *part* therapeutic commonality. Another way of conceiving this is to see the two of them as nuns and nurses, where nuns (akin to Shulmedizin doctors and 'ordained' to have a direct link to God, and best exemplified by the German epithet for doctors as 'Half-God in White') can be nurses and do all that nurses can do by training as nurses, while nurses (Heilpraktikers, not ordained and trained in the ways of God) may only be nurses. Like nurses, Heilpraktikers are excluded by law and training from the portals of Schulmedizin, except in so far as they have to know enough to 'do no harm' to the patient, and refer the patient to a Schulmedizin doctor where 'warranted'. This in fact is what the exam and viva voce are primarily for. This leaves the Heilpraktikers, who are not formally trained to practise any system of medicine, to fill their 'null set' by one or several therapeutic modalities of their choice. Since they are excluded from the portals of Schulmedizin, they willy-nilly fill this null set largely with a host of 'alternative' therapeutic possibilities as this is the training that is available to them. This happens either in special schools that train them to both pass their exam and train in different therapeutic systems, (for example, for five years in the case of Traditional Chinese Medicine) or through week-end or week-long programmes of 'continuing education', that they may share with Schulmedizin doctors.

It is thus evident that Heilpraktikers are a part homologue to the German Kur. While the Kur is alternative elsewhere and part of orthodox practice in Germany, similarly, alternative practices elsewhere are widely practised by Schulmedizin doctors and by legally licensed Heilpraktikers. It is only a part homologue as while the Kur is a medical specialisation, the Heilpraktiker is outside its ambit but legally competes in part with the Schulmedizin doctor. That the Heilpraktiker is unique to the West German therapeutic landscape is clear from the history of the Heilpraktiker by Unschuld, where he sketches its legal death by 1964 in East Germany and its virtual abortion in France as early as 1941 (Gaudillière 2010).

In the light of this the fact that the Heilpraktiker should practise several therapies should now come as no surprise as he is, among other things, filling that null set with what is available, without necessarily implying that they are a random selection. But the fact that Schulmedizin doctors also learn and deploy a host of these therapies is indeed surprising and calls for an explanation, which might in fact reciprocally and partially explain what the Heilpraktiker does. This is best done by returning to the ethnographic present and to the Heilpraktiker the paper began with, to look at a class of virtual patients.

Of relics, body parts and laser beams: virtual patients and cyber therapy

The Heilpraktiker, it transpired, had a whole class of patients who never arrived. Or rather, they arrived by post as little body parts: as a lock of hair or as drops of blood on blotting paper. The Heilpraktiker placed these body parts in the metal canister and wrapped the headphones around them and then proceeded to do exactly what was described earlier with the 'real' patient at the beginning of the paper. He then removed these body parts and placed the homeopathic sugar pills in the same canister, which were 'irradiated' through the laser beam with the simulated therapy; and these pills, instead of being necked with a band and handed over to the patient, were put in an envelope and dispatched to the patient by post. In other words, patients arrived by post and their medicines in turn arrived at their doorstep by post.

Patients who had thus arrived by post now constituted a library of body parts that had been duly catalogued and were readily retrievable. These readily retrievable patients in absentia, telephoned the Heilpraktiker when they were subsequently in trouble. He retrieved their body parts from the library, placed them in the canister, diagnosed them, and then proceeded to irradiate these body parts directly with the simulated therapy. In this last instance the therapy, rather than being dispatched to them as irradiated sugar pills, was beamed through cyberspace to the patient who was often still on the telephone. Or was it? After all the patient as synecdoche was indeed present in the canister, not metaphorically but literally as a body part, quite like the relics of saints – bones, nails, locks of hair and drops of blood on shrouds – found throughout Germany and the Catholic world, which the devout touched and whose (living?) presence served as the most palpable and material intercessory for the faithful. And at the other pole, did not such body parts, as part of conventional medical practice, also arrive by post as blood in vials at distant laboratories, or as locks of hair to test for mercury poisoning in tooth fillings?

While the ITA scan was thus central to this techno-sacramentalism, deployed as it was on the first and last day of 'real' incoming and exiting patients at the spa, there were other forms of techno-sacramentalism and scaramentals that the Heilpraktiker deployed and dispensed. What the practitioner did immediately after the ITA scan on the last day with an exiting patient was to open a wooden box of Bach's flower essences. He placed it on his lap, held aloft a conical metal pendulum suspended from a metal chain, and invited the patient to place her left forefinger on the first bottle and then 'doused' the pendulum. The dousing – what seemed like a little shake of the pendulum – produced a series of 'yes' and 'no' responses and resulted in the bottle being turned on its head for every yes and the patient skipping to the next bottle in case of a no. He then turned to a machine with a slot for a card like a credit card and a number of buttons. He inserted a card into the slot and then punched as many buttons as the number of essences chosen. After a brief moment he removed the card from the machine and gave it to the patient. Patients invariably and immediately held the card to their nose to smell the essence only to discover that there was no smell. They were then told that on the reverse side the flower essences were encoded on a magnetic strip. These pale purple cards with a small square hole meant for a string, were meant to be worn for about six weeks around the neck and against the skin, through which the encoded flower essences would seep through. Some of the patients carried this smart card in their purse; and some others slipped them into their brassiere. In one instance one of the patients, who was suffering from a grave auto-immune disorder (lupus erythematodes), when offered this smart card, pulled out a glass cube from her pocket, and subsequently over lunch told the author that the glass cube was an energy cube and that this was the one instance where she felt that the Heilpraktiker had addressed her emotions and her soul and not merely her body as the encoded flower essences, 'chosen' by the patients, seemed to answer their individual needs, such as making restless patients calm, selfish ones into loving and giving ones, and helped insomniacs to sleep. This particular patient had, apart from the two-week Ayurvedic regimen (primarily body therapies in her assessment), undergone virtually every diagnostic procedure and therapy in his armoury, ranging from the ITA scan, to Kirlian photography, to the dousing and the smart card, to being re-infused with her oxygenated blood, to homeopathic injections, to mushrooms, to a Japanese body touching exercise and yoga. But it was clear that either all her 'needs' were not met or she did not feel fully 'protected' by this panoply, as she wanted to know from the author – the Indian – as to whether she could find an Indian Guru on the internet; how she was headed next to the Egyptian pyramids as a therapeutic possibility; and before that she was going to send money, at the prompting of another patient, to a temple in India where a *homa*[12] would be performed for her welfare.

The panoply as a sign of a malaise and a cure

If it was earlier indicated why the Heilpraktiker was a poly-therapist, in so far as he was filling a null set, and filling it in on occasion in bits and pieces through week-end training programs, it is also possible to argue that the palette on offer was prompted by the possibility of so many small additions on the bill, quite like pizza toppings, where the pizza base in this case was Ayurveda. Another Heilpraktiker, when asked as to what prompted her to practise so many different therapies, said that many of them were like flavours that one sprinkled on a base. But many of these therapies, she said, gave her as a practitioner a deep sense of satisfaction like say colonic irrigation, which she had to stop doing after her two children came along, as it was both time consuming (time is money) and sapped her by its intensity.

A similar phenomenon is observed within the practice of Schulmedizin, where German doctors in their waiting lounges advertise for a wide range of Schulmedizin tests not covered by social or even private insurance, but which are supposedly near mandatory for the patient's welfare (such as special kind of breast scan for cancer; or a special 3D scan for a root canal that would minimise pain). Many patients are persuaded by this and pay out of pocket to the doctor. As an extension of this phenomenon is the increasing practice of offering 'alternative' therapies by Schulmedizin doctors, supposedly prompted by eliciting out of pocket payments or aimed at patients with private insurance (this of course would not be the doctor's point of view). While this economic motive is indeed an important explanatory strand in accounting for this phenomenon, and explains in part (some would argue a large part) why both Heilpraktikers and Schulmedizin doctors may be poly-therapists, and especially so in the context of the rather complex German health care system, it does not exhaust other explanatory possibilities. These other possibilities have, rather allusively and through a detour, been repeatedly signalled as constituting another explanatory strand: a strand that focuses on what the panoply may do for both patient and practitioner as both a therapeutic need and a meaning system, which as pointed out in the beginning is a fallout of a particular kind of epistemic impasse that Schulmedizin often finds itself in.

For example, the patient who had prompted the lupus patient to have a *homa* performed in India, recounted how her several years of torment had to come to an end a few days ago. She had been plagued by continuous twitching in various parts of her body, but especially her legs, and she had gone from pillar to post and had been run through the entire gamut of possibilities from a purely somatic diagnosis and surgery, to a 'soft in the head' diagnosis and psychiatry. She virtually broke down with both enormous relief and anger during this act of recounting, by saying that the Heilpraktiker had told her that there was nothing wrong with either her body or her head and the twitching was merely indicative of her constitutional type. This diagnosis was buttressed by another patient, an orthopaedist and an Ayurveda practitioner among other things, who confirmed this diagnosis and taught her some postural and breathing exercises.

Yet another patient who was there for a long-standing auto-immune disorder with her eye, had also been similarly shunted between an ophthalmologist and a psycho-therapist for other perceived emotional distress. She too, like the patient with the twitch, turned up there after having diligently saved her birthday and Christmas gifts over the last two years. At an average cost of €2500 for a 10 to 14 day stay, depending on the number of procedures prescribed and negotiated between patient and practitioner, an Ayurvedic Kur was not cheap for this predominantly non-wealthy clientele of school teachers, office assistants, salesgirls, and other Heilpraktikers. Since they had to pay out of pocket, what brought them there was often deep seated and long-standing issues with their being for which they had not found a solution with the Schulmedizin doctors, who divided their being into soma and psyche and further compounded this by parcelling out the somatic into different body parts and different disciplines leading often to an irreparable cognitive breakdown between practitioner and patient and thus propelling them in other directions.

The fact that this is part of a universal register is captured by Lawrence Kirmayer's (2000) 'Broken narratives', where a young, shy, woman with a heightened sense of propriety is 'kicked upstairs' to the psychiatrist when the gastroenterologists are unable to find a somatic lesion for her gastritis. This failure to find a lesion and hence a failure to diagnose, compounded by the failure to treat her 'symptoms', propels her toward the psychiatrist. The psychiatrist, if the therapy is to proceed, has to get the young lady to admit that she indeed has a psychological and not a somatic problem, which in this case is presumably 'caused' by a failed affair with an inappropriate man that her mother had frowned upon. The long and short of this encounter, according to Kirmayer, is that the young lady resists this narrative, which if accepted may have all kinds of repercussions for her self-esteem, and unhappy with the occlusion of her somatic complaint and wary of being reduced to a 'psychological nut case' (and thus stigmatised), refuses to play ball and breaks off the encounter and thus the possibility of a 'common' (a euphemism for the doctor's) narrative. But Kirmayer does not pause to ask the question as to where do these patients go? If Kirmayer is read in conjunction with Rhodes et al. (1999) and Naraindas (2006), one could argue that this kind of broken narrative is common-place and results in the case of patients walking out on the psychiatrist (as does the young lady in Kirmayer), or not going anywhere near one. Many of these patients then proceed, as Rhodes et al. (1999) point out, in the case of lower back pain and the lack of a lesion, toward an alternative practitioner like a chiropractor (in the US), or as Naraindas (2006) has shown, toward an Ayurvedic doctor in India. While Rhodes et al. call for a more diffuse and less localised understanding of aetiology, that is easier said than done as the local lesion is the *sine qua non* of modern medicine and it is in the aberrant tissue that the seeming aporias of clinical medicine in its founding moment finds its apodictic form (Foucault 1973). This not only leads to 'the disappearance of the sick man from medical cosmology' (Jewson 1976) and the silencing of his testimony (Canguilhem 1978), but results in the rather strange paradox of there being patients without a disease, and disease without a patient, which medical anthropology rather uncritically theorised by calling the first illness and the second disease, thereby tacitly subscribing to a biomedical model of the world.

But patients are not simply mind or body and neither are they patients only if an apparatus (and a biomedical one) announces their pathology through a lesion. The phenomenology of their experience and hence their testimony is cardinal to them, resulting in their turn to alternative therapists where mind-body testimony (and as was the case with the lupus patient, their mind-body-emotion-spirit and soul testimony) and not their mind OR body testimony, is allowed full expression; and for whom pain (the local site) is not the sign of a local lesion, whose absence delegitimises their pain and suffering, but the disease itself. It is this that leads Canguilhem (1978) to remark that pain is not in nature's plan; and pain is 'pain-disease' to be addressed in its own right. This 'pain-disease', as Naraindas (2006) has argued, the alternative therapist readily addresses, as his medicine either may not make this distinction or if it does its fault lines may be differently drawn, leading to a different conception of what constitutes 'the body'; and in any case it usually is an encounter where the somatic lesion is not the privileged point of origin and cause of disease (Naraindas 2006). Rather, as is the case with eighteenth-century European medicine, it is the testimony of her condition that is often the point of departure and this testimony may find other resolutions based on other theoretical frames, like the stretching and soft tissue work by an osteopath, after the orthopaedic has thrown up his arms as the X-ray, of say a knee, drew a blank.

Hence, itinerant patients are partly born of this epistemic impasse at the heart of Schulmedizin, which in turn has a bearing on how medical provisioning is arranged, resulting as it does in a particular kind of conversation between different systems or therapeutic styles. Many Schulmedizin doctors, fully aware of this impasse, either (often through a conversion experience that is gradual, or through a moment of epiphany) turn fully to other therapeutic formats, or seek to incorporate them piece-meal to augment what they see as a limitation of their practice; while for the Heilpraktikers, having been denied entry into the portals of Schulmedizin, this is indeed the raison d'être of their practice.

With this as the backdrop of why both Schulmedizin doctors and Heilpraktikers are poly-therapists, and how their panoply is a symptom of both a malaise and a cure born of a particular kind of epistemic impasse, one can now turn to the pizza base of the Heilpraktiker, namely the Ayurveda Kur, of which little has been said so far.

German Ayurveda as Pancakarma Kur

Without standing in judgement of whether Ayurveda in Germany is authentic or inauthentic, and how the Pancakarma (five cleansing procedures of the emesis, the enema, the purge, nasal errhines and bloodletting) has been either locally adapted or transformed, this paper advances the argument that the Ayurvedic spa is essentially built around a particular regimen, quite like the regimen that is characteristic of a Kur, and that this regimen is the Pancakarma, fashioned in a particular form that is German and in fact global. It appears at first instance that Pancakarma outside India is formatted and made the public face of Ayurveda. This is best exemplified by Deepak Chopra, who in a video shown to the patients at the spa, said that Ayurveda in the US is called Pancakarma Ayurveda or PK Ayurveda or just PK. In Germany, this becomes Pancakarma Kur, with websites that advertise it not only in Germany but for Germans who travel to have an Ayurveda Kur in Sri Lanka or India. This is borne out by the fact that most patients described the two to three week sojourn as an Ayurveda Kur, and once they come to terms with its modality called it a Pancakarma Kur, which in the dozen or so places visited (including some in Sri Lanka) was roughly similar.

Ayurvedic spas may be classified in various ways, with expensive ones where one dresses for an elaborate and posh dinner, and severe ones like the Heilpraktiker's spa, where patients did not dress for dinner, but came instead with towels wrapped around their head to virtually no dinner. Although set in a small pretty village, the place had nothing to offer patients by way of distraction. The food was spartan with virtually gruel for breakfast and dinner with the only hot meal being served at about noon which consisted of rice, lentils and vegetables, and only a rice gruel or 'conjee' for those under certain kinds of treatment.

Patients on arrival were broadly classified, at the end of an initial hour long consultation, into the three 'humoural' types as vata, pitta and kapha, with most of them being classified as vata. The outward institutionalisation of this classification was embodied in the three kinds of tea available round the clock, with vata tea being the most popular. This classification apart, a schedule of treatment was drawn up for the entire duration of the stay, a schedule that was often negotiated during the first consultation between patient and practitioner with cost being a major consideration. This daily schedule, which looked like a school timetable, included treatment and appropriate diet, and a more or less mandatory walk after lunch and dinner led by the Heilpraktiker at a brisk pace through the village, followed by a talk or demonstration after dinner in the foyer. The regimen, which started at day break and ended at about sunset, kept the patients on a constant treadmill, although it was probably not as demanding as the productive form of pleasure that Mackaman describes in the nineteenth-century French spa, where 'very early mornings were the rule at most baths...and...daily curing began with the drinking of mineral waters' (1998, 3). The Ayurvedic spa 'replaces' the early morning drinking of water by the drinking of 6 o'clock ghee (liquid clarified butter) and substitutes the mineral water by ginger water that patients are encouraged to drink till about noon. These increasing quantities of ghee (50, 100 and 150 ml) was a descent into purgatory, destined, through the complicated set of therapeutic procedures that followed, to purge the patients of their 'venial sins'. These procedures were literally versions of purging the patient of the vitiated doshas (humours), which in popular parlance is called detoxification (or detox for short). Patients complained bitterly and often re-enacted the 'ritual' by firmly pinching their nostrils and throwing their head back to indicate how they had gone through with it. Three days of ghee was the standard prelude and was part of the *purvakarmas* (preparatory regimen) that oleated the inside. This was followed by an external oleation, (popularly called the 'oil massage'), and then a sudation (either by sweating, or fomentation with herbal poultices, or a simply a hot shower), after which one or several of the Pancakarmas were administered.

It is instructive that invariably two of these procedures – emesis and blood letting – were usually not administered. They were supplanted instead by various dharas ('pouring' of oil over all or parts of the body), with the iconic among them being the shirodhara, where oil was streamed over the forehead through a long wicker from the bottom of a vessel. The vessel was made to swing back and forth over the forehead in a continuous pendulum-like motion, putting most patients to near sleep, or in terms of their own testimony, into a trance like condition. For most patients this state was not only immensely pleasurable but often had profound implications in so far as they seemed to 'find themselves' little by little, having, as they said, lost themselves in the quotidian act of living. In extreme cases they had 'out of body' experiences, moving them to write, sometimes in verse, of their experience. But in a small minority of cases it was experienced as being very unpleasant. For one gentleman in another spa, who seemed to be there primarily to humour his much younger partner, the shirodhara was almost unbearable as he began to relive his traumatic adolescence of the bombing of his town by allied forces, as the spa was situated not far from his childhood home. In either case the shirodhara, by common consent of both practitioners and patients, both in their private testimonies and in collective talk either in the tea room or over dinner, was described as Ayurvedic psychotherapy, where the analyst and the analysand was the patient.

While it is moot as to whether this was one of the intended effects of the shirodhara in the classical texts, or as practised in India for Indian patients, and how what may have been an obscure (and specific) procedure has now become the iconic commodity and public face of Global Ayurveda for Europeans and soon to follow middle class Indians, the fact remains that it seems to occasion an act of communing with the self by the patients. This communing and finding the self (although this may not always happen), occasioned by procedures like the shirodhara, or by the repeated hour-long massages with generous amounts of oil, was in fact a central motif in patient testimony, especially toward the end of their stay. Initial testimonies, on the contrary, were often mixed and sometimes the first shirodhara, for first time patients, brought on panic attacks, bringing them close to abandoning the spa. Long hours spent with them on a daily basis revealed that most patients, who were predominantly women, were there due to acute stress born of work and homemaking and a longstanding disease condition that had not found satisfactory resolution. This was often compounded by a life-cycle event like having tended to an ailing mother and often easing her into the nether world after a terminal illness; or, for the younger women, in their 40s, it was the ubiquitous broken relationship, which should rightfully be recognised and added to the repertoire of life-cycle events like birth, marriage and death, as it seems to have acquired a central place in the experience of a modern biography. Thus, apart from the therapeutic effects of the Pancakarma per se, or curing patients by offering them a different diagnosis, or making longstanding arthritic patients mobile and pain free, what the Kur seemed to do, notwithstanding a preamble or procedure that was painful, was to sink the patient into a kind of introspection.

Hence, beneath the seeming sybaritic exterior of patients sun bathing in lounge chairs after an oil massage, and without denying that pleasure and leisure were intrinsic to a spa experience, the Ayurvedic procedures and their aftermath, like waiting quietly in the room for two hours after an oil massage before a shower, led people to 'connect with their lost selves'. While this particular village had nothing by way of distraction, even in another spa, which had a lot of distractions, patients slowly withdrew into themselves, leading many of them to find a resolution to the psycho-socio-somatic condition that had propelled them there. The other side of this introspective journey was the substitute family of fellow sufferers and the sharing of experience, which also contributed to the healing. What was informal here was formalised in another Kur (which is the subject of another paper) for psycho-somatic patients, where patients were put together in batches of 11 people that would constitute the substitute 'family' and a fully theorised therapeutic resource.

The Kur as a fusion of the sybaritic and the therapeutic

While it is evident that the Kur thus allows the patients to recover and rehabilitate themselves, it is important to note that all the therapeutic procedures, rather than being conceived as merely an aid to recovery, and without denying that they may indeed be an aid to recovery, may also be seen as directly addressing the patient's diseased condition. Hence, an 'oil massage' for example, within the theoretical framework of Ayurveda, may not merely be an aid but is a 'vata hara' or an antidote to vata, the humour (a contentious translation) responsible for a host of diseased conditions including body pain, restlessness, sleeplessness, impaired digestion, arthritis, etc. Further, if the oil massage is made a preamble to a karma (action), such as a vasti (enema), this preamble and the procedure, along with rest (also a vata hara) and an appropriate vata hara diet, function not as a mere 'aid' to recovery but as the precise mode of addressing the patient's disease. In this re-theorised framework, what appears sybaritic, or aids to recovery, turns out to be directly therapeutic and sometimes pleasurable.

The current re-classification of the Kur as Reha, or rehabilitation, however, militates against this possibility of the Kur as a cure and moves it toward the pole of wellness rather than medicine, wherein the Reha comes to be seen, like physiotherapy for example, as an adjunct to the practice of medicine. Only time will tell whether the Kur reinvents itself under the notion of Reha, and whether the boundaries between Wellness and the Reha and Kur in its dwindled form are made more watertight or fuzzy. While there are already emergent hybrids like Reha-Kur and Wellness-Kur, the Kur for the generation under 40 is among the best examples of how their parents' generation took advantage of social welfare during their working life and, to make it worse, retired early. This generation feel they are paying for their parents' long summer of retirement, and that their contribution to their future pension rather than cushioning their own future is immediately distributed to their parents, leading to 'the empty coffer syndrome'. This is the intergenerational accusation sometimes heard at dinner, much to the chagrin of the older generation, who in this narrative suddenly appear as vampires. Hence, for this generation, wellness with its connotation of fitness and holiday is welcome, and to be paid out of pocket, while the Kur, with its current connotation of self-indulgence and work shirking is out. But these are large narratives and difficult to generalise, and for those undergoing a Kur, usually women, and with an average age of 55, the Kur is viewed and experienced rather differently.

This essay, by examining the twin German institutions of the Kur and the Heilpraktiker, has led to an interrogation of the invidious distinctions between medicine and alternative medicine, or between cure and Kur, and between sybaritic and therapeutic forms. It transpires that the Kur and the Heilpraktiker, and the 'secret' practice of German Schulmedizin doctors who sometimes – if not frequently – practise medicine as if they were Heilpraktikers, are a testimony to a blurring of boundaries on the one hand and a drawing of boundaries on the other. What emerges from this blurring and drawing of boundaries is that in both the Kur and the practice of the Heilpraktiker, the fault lines between mind and body are either differently drawn or made fuzzy, although the formal categories of Schulmedizin impose themselves even here by dividing the Heilpraktikers themselves into 'small' Heilpraktikers who deal only with the 'mind' and do not prescribe drugs (like psychotherapists rather than psychiatrists) and the 'big' Heilpraktikers who deal with the 'body'. That this may not be the case in living practice is evident from the fact that the Heilpraktiker under study seems to address several facets of a person's being by his poly-therapeutics, including the emotional, the spiritual and the cosmic, that Schulmedizin attempts to keep apart, only to be brought in through the back door by the doctors themselves, or left to the Heilpraktikers to explore and experiment with their panoply of therapeutic possibilities. And it is evident that both healers and patients need this panoply now as much as they did in the past.

Acknowledgements

This paper owes a great deal to the warmth and generosity of the Heilpraktiker and the patients at the Spa. They both gave of their time, allowed the author to sit in on consultations, and readily shared a part of their life and being, often over extended conversations. Thanks are also due to the principal therapist at the spa, who also generously gave of his time. The research for this paper is part of a larger project at the University of Heidelberg and the author would like to thank all the collaborators of project C3, especially William Sax and Anand Samir Chopra; the SAI for being wonderful hosts, especially Manfred Hake and Martin Gieselman; and Laila, Anthony, Justus and Kinga for being good research assistants. The paper has benefited a great deal from the careful reading and comments from the referees, and from Nupur, Bo, Nina, and Katyayani.

Ethics and funding

This research was part of Project C3, Cluster of Excellence, Asia and Europe, at the University of Heidelberg; and the funding came through a Joint-Appointment Professorship at the South Asia Institute, Department of Anthropology, University of Heidelberg. Neither at Heidelberg nor at my parent university, the Jawaharlal Nehru University, is there a provision to have the project vetted through an Institutional Review Board. But since ethnography is a covenant, the general principles of ethnographic research were followed by asking the Heilpraktiker permission to conduct the study in writing. All the patients interviewed and observed at the spa were told, both by the author and the Heilpraktiker, why the author was there; and the purpose of the study was explained to the patients and their anonymity guaranteed. The names of interviewees are pseudonyms and the spa remains unidentified.
Conflict of interest: none.

Notes

1. The name of the scanning device has been changed so as not comment on the scan as a product, or the particular uses to which it can supposedly be put to, and the use made of it by the Heilpraktiker. For a survey on the nature of unconventional medicine in Europe see Aldridge (1994). For a study, in English, on the Heilpraktiker and their practice, see Demling (2002) and Demling et al. (2002). Between them, one can glean how widespread some of the therapies on offer with the Heilpraktiker are in Germany.
2. The late sixteenth-century roots of the word 'panoply' means a complete protection for spiritual warfare, although its current meaning merely means a 'complete or impressive collection of things'. As the essay unfolds, the current and common meaning will resonate with its 'older' meaning of a 'complete spiritual armoury'. (cf. the 'Panoply of God': Ephesians 6:13).
3. The German term of Schulmedizin, meaning those who have been formally trained in a university, may be a far better term than biomedicine. In any case, in the German context, it makes a perfect contrast to the praxis of the Heilpraktiker, and will be used when it seems warranted.
4. The case for the strict separation of the Reha, from the Kur and Wellness (clubbed together in opposition), is advocated in the latest issue of the Deutches Ärzteblatt, by Wirth et al. (2010). The Reha is a six billion dollar industry with 1200 centres recognized by the pension fund alone.
5. For the spa in the tropics, see Jennings (2006).
6. For an explication of this debate see Livingstone (1999).
7. This is a history that is waiting to be written. It is not surprising that it has not yet been written, given the current scepticism about water as a cure for anything at all, let alone smallpox.
8. Mud baths, traced in part to Paracelsus were made popular by Emanuel Felke (1856–1926) – the mud Pastor as he was called – and are also known as Felke baths.
9. The 'proof' of this admixture may well come from the fact that the spa industry is much larger in Germany than in France but only 50% of the cases are paid for by insurance, while in the smaller French spa industry, 90% are paid by social insurance and hence almost fully medicalised.
10. The difference, however, is that the Kur is potentially reimbursable by the statutory health insurance, although this has enormously dwindled; while these non-conventional therapies may be reimbursable only by additional private insurance.
11. The Germans seem to have a three-tiered class-based schooling system called the Hauptschule (9 years), which roughly produces/reproduces blue collar workers, the Realschule (10 years) that reproduces white collar workers and the gymnasium (13 years, and now 12 years) that sends students to the university. The children are sorted out into these three streams at about age 10.
12. A religious practice in Hinduism, Buddhism and Jainism, involving making offerings into a consecrated fire.

References

Aldridge, D. 1994. Unconventional medicine in Europe. *Advances: The Journal of Mind/Body Health* 10, no. 2: 1–7.
Boudin, J.C.H.M. 1856. *Traité de géographie et de statistique médicale des maladies épidémiques.* Paris: J.B. Bailliére.
Canguilhem, G. 1978. *On the normal and the pathological.* Boston: D. Riedel Publishing.
Cayleff, S.E. 1987. *Wash and be healed. The water-cure movement and women's health.* Philadelphia: Temple University Press.
Clark, J. 1830. *The influence of climate in the prevention and cure of chronic diseases, more particularly of the chest and digestive organs.* London: Thomas and George Underwood.
Davidson, A. 1892. *Geographical pathology: An inquiry into the geographical distribution of infective and climatic diseases.* London: Y. J. Pentland.

Demling, J.H. 2002. Heilpraktiker. *Complementary Therapies in Medicine* 10: 192.

Demling, J.H., S. Neubauer, H.-J. Luderer, and M. Wörthmüller. 2002. A survey on psychiatric patients' use of non-medical alternative practitioners: Incidence, methods, estimation, and satisfaction. *Complementary Therapies in Medicine* 10: 193–201.

Deutscher-heilbaederverband, 2010 http://www.deutscher-heilbaederverband.de/cms/pages/posts/bedeutung-der-deutschen-heilbaeder-und-Kurorte43.pHeilpraktiker (accessed 20 June 2010).

Floyer, J. 1702. *The ancient psykhroloysia* [Greek transliterated] *revived: or, an essay to prove cold bathing both safe and useful.* London: Sam. Smith and Benj. Walford.

Foucault, M. 1973. *The birth of the clinic: An archaeology of medical perception.* Trans. A.M. Sheridan Smith. London: Tavistock.

Gaudillière, J.P. 2010. Une marchandise scientifique? Savoirs, industrie et régulation du médicament dans L'Allemagne des années trente. *Annales HSS* Janvier-février, no. 1: 89–120.

Hamlin, Christopher. 1990. Chemistry, medicine, and the legitimization of English spas 1740–1840. In *The medical history of waters and spas*, ed. Roy Porter. *Medical History*, Supplement no. 10, 67–81.

Hancocke, J. 1722. *Febrifugum magnum: or, common water the best cure for fevers, and probably for the plague.* London: R. Halsey & J. Roberts.

Holwell, J.Z. 1767. An account of the manner of inoculating for the smallpox in the East Indies. In *Indian science and technology in the eighteenth century: Some contemporary British accounts*, ed. Dharampal, 195–218. Delhi: Impex India, 1983.

Jennings, Eric T. 2006. *Curing the Colonizers: Hydrotherapy, Climatology, and French Colonial Spas.* Durham: Duke University Press.

Jewson, N.D. 1976. The disappearance of the sick man from medical cosmology, 1770–1870. *Sociology* 10: 225–44.

Johnson, J. 1831. *Change of air, or the philosophy of traveling.* New York: Samuel Wood & Sons.

Kirmayer, L.J. 2000. Broken narratives: Clinical encounters and the poetics of illness experience. In *Narrative and the cultural construction of illness and healing*, ed. C. Mattingly and L. Garro, 153–80. Berkeley: University of California Press.

Livingstone, D.N. 1999. Tropical climate and moral hygiene: the anatomy of a Victorian debate. *The British Journal for the History of Science* 32, no. 1: 93–110.

Mackaman, D.P. 1998. *Leisure settings: Bourgeois culture, medicine, and the spa in modern France.* Chicago: University of Chicago Press.

Maretzki, T.W. 1987. The Kur in West Germany as an interface between naturopathic and allopathic ideologies. *Social Science and Medicine* 24: 1061–68.

Maretzki, T.W. 1989. Cultural variation in biomedicine: The Kur in West Germany. *Medical Anthropology Quarterly* 3, no. 1: 22–35.

Maretzki, T.W., and E. Seidler. 1985. Biomedicine and naturopathic healing in West Germany: A historical and ethnomedical view of a stormy relationship. *Culture, Medicine and Psychiatry* 9: 383–421.

Naraindas, H. 1996. Poisons, putrescence and the weather: A genealogy of the advent of tropical medicine. *Contributions to Indian Sociology* 30, no. 1: 1–35.

Naraindas, H. 2003. Preparing for the pox: A theory of smallpox in Bengal and Britain. *Asian Journal of Social Sciences* 31, no. 2: 304–39.

Naraindas, H. 2006. Of spineless babies and folic acid: Evidence and efficacy in biomedicine and Ayurvedic medicine. Special issue, *Social Science and Medicine* 62, no. 11: 2658–69.

Rhodes, L., C. McPhillips-Tangum, C. Markham, and R. Klenk. 1999. The power of the visible: The meaning of diagnostic tests in chronic back pain. *Social Science and Medicine* 48: 1189–203.

Speier, A. 2011. Health tourism in a Czech spa. *Anthropology and Medicine* 18, no. 1: 55–66.

Thornton, F., and H. Brutscher. 2009. What is a spa? Historical background and modern influences. http://spas.about.com/ (accessed 20 December 2009).

Thorowgood, J.C. 1868. *The climatic treatment of consumption and chronic lung diseases.* London: H. K. Lewis.

Unschuld, P. 1980. The issue of structured coexistence of scientific and alternative medical systems: A comparison of East and West German legislation. *Social Science and Medicine* 14B: 5–24.

Weber, H., and G.M. Foster. 1896. *Climate in the treatment of disease.* Vol. 1 of *A system of medicine*, ed. C.T. Albutt, 247–300. London: Macmillan.

Weisz, G. 2001. Spas, mineral waters, and hydrological science in twentieth-century France. *Isis* 92, no. 3: 451–83.

Wirth, A., G. Klein, and H-J. Lepthin. 2010. Medizinische Rehabilitation. Bessere Vernetzung notwendig. *Deutsches Ärzteblatt, Jg.* 107, no. 25: 1253–6.

Globalization and gametes: reproductive 'tourism,' Islamic bioethics, and Middle Eastern modernity

Marcia C. Inhorn

Department of Anthropology, Yale University,
New Haven, CT, USA

'Reproductive tourism' has been defined as the search for assisted reproductive technologies (ARTs) and human gametes (eggs, sperm, embryos) across national and international borders. This article conceptualizes reproductive tourism within 'global reproscapes,' which involve the circulation of actors, technologies, money, media, ideas, and human gametes, all moving in complicated manners across geographical landscapes. Focusing on the Muslim countries of the Middle East, the article explores the Islamic 'local moral worlds' informing the movements of Middle Eastern infertile couples. The ban on third-party gamete donation in Sunni Muslim-majority countries and the recent allowance of donor technologies in the Shia Muslim-majority countries of Iran and Lebanon have led to significant movements of infertile couples across Middle Eastern national borders. In the new millennium, Iran is leading the way into this 'brave new world' of high-tech, third-party assisted conception, with Islamic bioethical discourses being used to justify various forms of technological assistance. Although the Middle East is rarely regarded in this way, it is a key site for understanding the intersection of technoscience, religious morality, and modernity, all of which are deeply implicated in the new world of reproductive tourism.

Introduction

What motivates the global movements of infertile people searching for new reproductive technologies and human gametes? Inspired by recent developments in globalization theory, medical anthropology, gender studies, and science and technology studies, this article focuses on the newly described phenomenon of 'reproductive tourism,' also known as 'fertility tourism,' 'procreative tourism,' and 'cross-border reproductive care' (CBRC). Reproductive tourism is defined as 'the traveling by candidate service recipients from one institution, jurisdiction or country where treatment is not available to another institution, jurisdiction or country where they can obtain the kind of medically assisted reproduction they desire. As such, it is part of the more general "medical tourism"' (Pennings 2002, 337).

Little is known about the motivations of reproductive tourists in any part of the world. A front-page story in *The New York Times* on January 25, 2005, entitled 'Fertility Tourists Go Great Lengths to Conceive,' claimed that infertile Americans were seeking services abroad, 'in places like South Africa, Israel, Italy, Germany, and Canada, where the costs can be much lower' (Lee 2005, A1). However, economic factors may not be the sole consideration. Scholars who are beginning to theorize the relationship between nation-states, reproductive tourism, and global reproductive rights suggest that the causes of such transnational tourism may be manifold. Eight discrete, but often interrelated, factors promoting reproductive tourism have been cited in the existing literature: (1) individual countries may prohibit a specific service for religious or ethical reasons; (2) a specific service may be unavailable because of lack of expertise, equipment, or lack of donor gametes (eggs, sperm or embryos); (3) a service may be unavailable because it is not considered sufficiently safe or its risks are unknown, so that countries exercising safety precautions may prohibit procedures that are available elsewhere; (4) certain categories of individuals may not receive a service, especially at public expense, on the basis of age, marital status, or sexual orientation; (5) services operate on a market or quasi-market basis, particularly in relation to donor gametes, thus affecting both affordability and supply (including shortages and waiting lists); (6) services may simply be cheaper in other countries; (7) patients may have concerns about low-quality medical services; and finally, (8) privacy concerns may lead some patients to travel (Blyth and Farrand 2005; Deech 2003; Pennings 2002).

These 'causes' of reproductive tourism are still speculative, as little empirical research has yet to be undertaken. Yet, even in the absence of empirical data, a policy debate is growing over the desirability of national and international legislation to restrict reproductive tourism. As Penning notes in *The Journal of Medical Ethics*, 'The more widespread this phenomenon, the louder the call for international measures to stop these movements' (Pennings 2002, 337).

Most of the extant literature on reproductive tourism focuses on the West, particularly upon border-crossing between European Union nations (Storrow 2005). Little is known about reproductive tourism outside of Euro-America, or about the forces that motivate infertile persons to undertake international travel in their 'quests for conception' (Inhorn 1994). Only through in-depth, ethnographic analysis of the actual stories, desires, and migratory pathways of reproductive tourists themselves may scholars begin to shed light on the complex calculus of factors governing this global movement of reproductive actors.

This article examines the theoretical interplay between forces of globalization and reproductive tourism in the Middle East. It will begin with Arjun Appadurai's theory of global 'scapes,' which is highly relevant and useful in thinking about the global landscape in which assisted reproductive technologies (ARTs) are being rapidly deployed. But, Appadurai's work needs to be 'engendered' and expanded to include the complex 'reproscape' in which the multiple 'flows' of reproductive tourism occur. In the global reproscape, issues of bodily commodification are paramount, given that reproductive tourism may be undertaken explicitly to procure human gametes, both sperm and eggs, which are disassociated from men's and women's bodies and increasingly sold on the open market. Furthermore, the language of reproductive 'tourism' itself comes into question when the subjectivities of reproductive travelers themselves are taken into consideration. In short, a whole new vocabulary is needed to represent the global flows and scapes surrounding ARTs in the new millennium.

The second half of the article turns to the author's empirical work on reproductive tourism in the Muslim Middle East, based on ethnographic research that was carried out there over the past 20 years, and particularly since the year 2003.[1] As will be argued, reproductive 'tourism' in the Middle East is inflected by local moral attitudes toward science, technology, and medicine, and particularly varying Islamic bioethical positions on the donation of human gametes. Furthermore, the implications of gamete donation for marriage, kinship, and gender relations are tremendous, perhaps especially for infertile Muslim couples. But first, it is important to situate this topic of reproductive tourism – and the search for human gametes in the Middle East – within the broader theoretical literature on globalization and specifically global flows.

Globalization and reproductive tourism: theorizing reproscapes

Globalization can be understood, in a most basic sense, 'as the ever faster and ever denser streams of people, images, consumer goods, money markets, and communication networks around the world' (Schaebler and Stenberg 2004, xv–xvi). Anthropologists have contributed significantly to theorizing the nature of these global flows, and to providing numerous ethnographic examples of the 'glocal,' or the reception of things 'global' at various 'local' levels (Appadurai 1996; Basch, Glick Schiller, and Blanc 1994; Friedman 1994; Hannerz 1996; Inhorn 2003; Lewellen 2002; Ong and Collier 2005; Ritzer 2002).

One of the major anthropological theorists of globalization, Arjun Appadurai, has delineated a 'global cultural economy' in which global movements operate through five pathways, which he famously calls 'scapes' (Appadurai 1990, 1996). According to Appadurai, globalization is characterized by the movement of people (ethnoscapes), technology (technoscapes), money (financescapes), images (mediascapes), and ideas (ideoscapes), which now follow increasingly complex trajectories, moving at different speeds across the globe. Appadurai reminds us that this transnational movement of people, goods, and ideas is both a deeply historical and inherently localizing process. In other words, globalization is not enacted in a uniform manner around the world, nor is it simply culturally homogenizing in its effects.

The phenomenon of reproductive tourism clearly involves two of Appadurai's five scapes – namely, ethnoscapes and technoscapes. Ethnoscapes, according to Appadurai (1996, 33), involve 'the landscape of persons who constitute the shifting world in which we live: tourists, immigrants, refugees, exiles, guest workers, and other moving groups and individuals.' Technoscapes involve 'the global configuration, also ever fluid, of technology and the fact that technology, both high and low, both mechanical and informational, now moves at high speeds across various kinds of previously impervious boundaries' (Appadurai 1996, 34).

However, a consideration of reproductive tourism has the potential to expand upon Appadurai's theory of globalization. Despite the heuristic appeal of five discrete global scapes, one scape of significant medical anthropological interest – namely, the 'bioscape' of moving biological substances and body parts – might be added to Appadurai's list.[2] Using Appadurai's language of 'scapes,' reproductive tourism might be thought of productively as a more complex 'reproscape' – a kind of 'meta-scape' combining numerous dimensions of globalization and global flows. To wit, reproductive tourism occurs in a new world order characterized not only by circulating reproductive technologies (technoscapes), but also by circulating reproductive actors (ethnoscapes) and their gametes (bioscapes), leading to a large-scale global industry (financescapes), in which images (mediascapes) and ideas (ideoscapes) about making lovely babies while 'on holiday' come into play. This reproscape entails a distinct geography traversed by global flows of reproductive actors, technologies, body parts, money, and reproductive imaginaries (e.g., the birth of 'miracle' babies).

Furthermore, this reproscape is highly gendered – with technologies enacted on men's and women's bodies in highly differentiated ways. Gender was never the focus of Appadurai's original work on globalization. Yet, the ethnoscape of moving peoples, the technoscape of moving technologies, the bioscape of moving body parts, and the ideoscape of moving procreative scenarios are, indeed, highly gendered, and this is a feature of globalization that must be analyzed. Reproscapes also entail new forms of reproductive labor among reproductive 'assistors,' who, in many cases are women, and who undergo risky forms of hormonal stimulation and oocyte (egg) harvesting. However, reproductive assistance also has the potential to create kin-like female alliances, including between actual kin who donate their oocytes to relatives, as well as between unrelated women who 'share' their oocytes with other women in infertility clinics or donate them for a fee. Oocyte donation in particular invokes the notion of altruistic 'gift exchange' between women, even though oocytes are increasingly sold on the reproductive marketplace for up to $50,000, especially for 'Ivy League' oocytes of presumed superior intelligence and other ineffable qualities. Indeed, the very language of 'reproductive assistance' is called into question, when assistance comes at such a high cost.

In addition, to use the language of 'reproductive tourism' to define this field of global flows is a bit of a misnomer (Inhorn and Patrizio 2009). It is important to note that, in some countries, 'clinics that cater to fertility tourists appear to welcome the development of new markets and have undertaken to market their services so as to create a fantasy of conceiving a child during a romantic holiday' (Storrow 2005, 326–327). But is overseas test-tube baby-making a holiday? In his excellent theoretical analysis of reproductive tourism, legal theorist Richard Storrow (2005) questions the trope of 'tourism' as an appropriate gloss for fertility travel. As he notes, tourism is a type of traveling that involves leisure, pleasure, and free time. Fertility tourism, on the other hand, is quite a different story:

> Fertility tourism occurs when infertile individuals or couples travel abroad for the purposes of obtaining medical treatment for their infertility. Fertility tourism may also occur in the reverse, when the infertile import the third parties necessary for their fertility treatment. These definitions of fertility tourism are, on the one hand, difficult to harmonize with the idea of tourism as pleasure travel, particularly given that some infertile individuals describe their condition as devastatingly painful and their effort to relieve it as requiring enormous physical and emotional exertion (Storrow 2005, 300).

More neutral terms, such as 'reproductive travel' or 'cross-border reproductive care' are beginning to enter the clinical lexicon (Inhorn and Patrizio 2009). However, the use of the term 'reproductive exile' more accurately captures the feelings and experiences of many infertile couples who feel 'forced' to travel to seek ART assistance across borders. Indeed, the term 'tourism' must be avoided, for it can never fully capture the stories of travel and hardship experienced by the infertile in their border crossings. The term 'tourism' will be dispensed with in the remainder of this article.

Moreover, the notion of 'stratified reproduction,' forwarded by medical anthropologists Faye Ginsburg and Rayna Rapp (1995), evokes the transnational inequalities whereby some well-to-do infertile couples are able to achieve their reproductive desires, including through resort to reproductive technologies and reproductive travel, while other infertile couples of lesser means are disempowered and even despised as reproducers. Only 48 of the 191 member states of the World Health Organization offer ARTs to their citizens, with less than 1% of the projected needs for ARTs met in the largest countries of the world (China, India, Pakistan, Indonesia, Egypt) (Inhorn 2009). In these countries, the average cost of one cycle of IVF exceeds the average income of half the population, making ARTs easily affordable only for elites (Inhorn 2003). In other words, the global 'reproscape' in which reproductive tourism takes place is an uneven terrain, in that some individuals, some communities, and some nations have achieved greater access to the fruits of reproductive globalization than others. The term 'stratified reproscape' might be added to the lexicon to describe the unevenness of ART access around the world.[3]

In the author's earlier studies of in vitro fertilization in Egypt, which were characterized as a 'quest for conception' (Inhorn 1994), she examined numerous local barriers to ART access, calling these 'arenas of constraint,' or the structural, ideological, social relational, and practical obstacles and apprehensions that constrain and sometimes prohibit altogether the uses of ARTs (Inhorn 2003). More than a decade later, little is known about the various arenas of constraint that face infertile couples in their 'transnational quests for conception.'

However, one of the major prohibitions cited by legal scholars who have written about reproductive tourism is the prohibition on access to human gametes (Blyth and Farrand 2005; Deech 2003; Pennings 2002). Several Western nations, including Italy, Norway, Canada, and Great Britain, have enacted strict legislation prohibiting some or all forms of gamete donation, especially anonymous gamete donation, as well as gestational surrogacy. Such restrictions have triggered European fertility tourism on a massive scale, mostly of infertile Western Europeans to the 'white' post-Soviet bloc of Eastern Europe (such as Russia, Slovenia, and Romania). There, clinics can 'employ the Internet to attract fertility tourists with promises of cut-rate in vitro fertilization, high success rates, liberal reproductive policies and little administrative oversight' (Storrow 2005, 307). Furthermore, young women in these countries may comprise a vulnerable population of egg donors, who are compelled out of economic necessity to sell their eggs in the local reproductive marketplace (Storrow 2005). Given the newly recognized category of the 'traveling foreign egg donor' who seeks economic mobility through the sale of her body parts (Heng 2007), Storrow points to the parallels between unregulated fertility tourism and sex tourism, as young women in the economically deteriorated post-communist societies discover that prostitution and egg donation offer economic rewards. As Storrow (2005, 327) argues, 'egg donation, like prostitution, will be especially attractive in regions of the world where large numbers of women with few choices want to improve their economic circumstances by any means available.'

Indeed, 'bodily commodification' – namely, selling gametes and other body parts for the purposes of reproduction and medical research – has become one of the major areas of study in both medical anthropology and science and technology studies (Cohen 1999, 2002; Lock 2001; Scheper-Hughes 2000, 2002a, 2002b; Sharp 2000, 2006). Bodily penetration, fragmentation, and commodification are clearly operative in the world of assisted reproduction, a world that has evolved dramatically since the birth of Louise Brown, the world's first 'test-tube baby,' in 1978. Since then, the invention of in vitro fertilization (IVF) to overcome female infertility has paved the way for:

- intracytoplasmic sperm injection (ICSI) to overcome male infertility;
- third-party gamete donation (of eggs, sperm, embryos, and uteruses, as in surrogacy) to overcome absolute sterility;
- multi-fetal pregnancy reduction to selectively abort high-order IVF pregnancies;
- ooplasm transfer (OT) to improve egg quality in perimenopausal women;
- cryopreservation, storage, and disposal of unused gametes and embryos;
- preimplantation genetic diagnosis (PGD) to select 'against' embryos with genetic defects and to select 'for' embryos of a specific sex;
- embryonic stem cell research on unused embryos for the purposes of therapeutic intervention; and
- the future possibility of asexual autonomous reproduction through human cloning.

With virtually all of these technologies, sperm and eggs are retrieved from bodies, embryos are returned to bodies, and sometimes they are donated to other bodies or used for the purposes of stem cell and other forms of medical research (Franklin 1996; Kahn 2000; Kirkman 2003; Konrad 1998). As noted earlier, ARTs exact a significant physical toll on the body, especially for women as both recipients of ARTs and as oocyte donors (Inhorn 2003, Kahn 2000; Lorber 1989; Storrow 2005; van der Ploeg 1995). Furthermore, despite the existence of national and international statements opposing the commercialization of ART services, significant commodification has occurred as gametes and embryos are increasingly sold on the open market through Internet websites and college newspapers (with such advertisements as 'Sperm Donors Needed – We Will Pay!') (Blank 1998; Braverman 2001; Carmeli and Birenbaum-Carmeli 2000; Pollock 2003; Shanley 2002; Thompson 2005). In her article on 'Reproductive Tourism in Europe,' Ruth Deech (2003, 425) questions the human rights implications of the documented massive global transfer within the European Union of sperm, eggs, and embryos 'passed from country to country in search of one that permits the desired treatment or allows the chosen gametes to be used.'

The Middle East is different from the EU countries in terms of its attitudes toward commodification and bodily transfer of human gametes. In the Middle East, an ART industry is flourishing, with hundreds of IVF clinics in countries ranging from the small Arab Gulf states to the larger but less prosperous nations of North Africa (Inhorn 2003; Serour 1996, 2008; Serour and Dickens 2001). This development of a mostly private Middle Eastern ART industry is not surprising: Islam encourages the use of science and medicine as solutions to human suffering and is a religion that can be described as 'pronatalist,' encouraging the growth of an Islamic 'multitude' (Brockopp 2003; Inhorn 1994; Musallam 1986).

Yet, relatively little is known about Islam and technoscience, if technoscience is defined broadly as the interconnectedness between science and technology through 'epistemological, institutional, and cultural discursive practices' (Lotfalian 2004, 1). As noted by Lotfalian (2004, 6) in his recent monograph on *Islam, technoscientific identities, and the culture of curiosity*, there is a glaring lacuna in the literature on science and technology in cross-cultural perspective, particularly from the Islamic world, where there are 'really only two strains of relevant work' – first, on the Islamic medieval sciences and, second, on philosophical arguments for civilizational differences between Islamic and Western science and technology. This dearth of relevant scholarship clearly applies to the cross-cultural study of ARTs. For example, in the second edition of the seminal volume on *Third party assisted conception across cultures: Social, legal and ethical perspectives* (Blyth and Landau 2004), not a single Muslim society is represented among the 13 country case studies.

Clearly, the time has come to examine the globalization of ARTs to diverse contexts in the Muslim world, particularly given the rapid development and deployment of these technologies. In addition to examining the ART 'technoscape,' it is equally important to examine the 'ethnoscape' of reproductive actors as they move across the Middle East. ARTs in the Middle East bespeak a complex reproscape of moving peoples, technologies, gametes, money, images, and ideas involving the pursuit of conception. That infertile couples are willing to participate in this Middle Eastern reproscape bespeaks the love, commitment, and ardent desire for children that characterize most couples in the Middle East, but which are rarely emphasized in the Western media discourses about the purported violence, fanaticism, and cruelty of Arab men to women (Inhorn 2007). As will be shown in the story of an infertile Syrian couple that follows, the romantic love and conjugal commitments between many infertile Muslim couples are fueling the IVF industry in the Middle East. Love, commitment, and the desire to become parents are also causing some couples to venture abroad in search of gametes.

The Middle Eastern reproscape: understanding Islamic local moral worlds

What motivates infertile Middle Eastern couples to travel overseas in search of ARTs? Although there are a wide variety of motivating factors behind reproductive travel (Inhorn and Shrivastav 2010), anthropologists and other scholars studying ARTs in the Middle East have called attention to Islam and the so-called 'local moral worlds' of Middle Eastern Muslim infertile couples. Indeed, nearly a dozen scholars are now participating in this scholarly endeavor (Inhorn and Tremayne, in press).

Arthur Kleinman (1995, 45) has called local moral worlds 'the commitments of social participants in a local world about what is at stake in everyday experience.' Understanding the rapidly evolving moral-religious climate surrounding ARTs in the Muslim world is imperative. To do so requires examining *fatwas*, or non-legally binding but authoritative religious decrees, as well as the subsequent ethical and legal rulings that are being issued to enforce or, in some cases, overturn these *fatwa* rulings (Inhorn and Tremayne, in press; Moosa 2003; Tremayne 2009). However, understanding local moral worlds also involves asking what Muslim ART-seekers think about IVF and specifically donor technologies. When faced with the need for donor gametes to overcome infertility, what do Muslim IVF patients do? Is the search for human gametes one of the major motivating factors for reproductive tourism in the Middle East, as suggested by the theoretical literature on this phenomenon? At this point, these questions provide compelling material for a study of what might be called 'technoscience in practice.'

As explained in the forthcoming volume *Islam and assisted reproductive technologies: Sunni and Shia perspectives* (Inhorn and Tremayne, forthcoming), major divergences in Islamic juridical opinion between Sunni and Shia religious authorities have led to striking differences in the practice of ARTs, particularly with regard to the use of donor gametes. These differences in practice have led to new local moral worlds among Muslim IVF patients, as well as new transnational reproflows across Middle Eastern borders. The differences in the dominant Sunni position on ARTs will be briefly described, before turning to Shia innovations that have had major moral and practical implications for Muslim couples in their quests for donor gametes.

Sunni Islam and IVF

To begin with Sunni Islam, the Grand Shaikh of Egypt's famed religious university, Al Azhar, issued the first *fatwa* on medically-assisted reproduction on March 23, 1980. This initial *fatwa* – issued only two years after Louise Brown's birth in England, but a full six years before the opening of Egypt's first IVF center – has proved to be truly authoritative and enduring in all its main points. In fact, the basic tenets of the original Al-Azhar *fatwa* on IVF have been upheld by other *fatwas* issued since 1980 in Egypt, Saudi Arabia, Malaysia, and beyond, thereby achieving wide acceptance across the Sunni Muslim world (Inhorn, Patrizio, and Serour, in press; Serour 2008).

The Sunni Islamic position on assisted reproduction clearly permits in vitro fertilization, using eggs from the wife with the sperm of her husband and the transfer of the fertilized embryos back to the uterus of the same wife. However, since marriage is a contract between the wife and husband during the span of their marriage, no third party should intrude into the marital functions of sex and procreation. This means that a third party donor is *not* acceptable, whether he or she is providing sperm, eggs, embryos, or a uterus (as in surrogacy). As noted by Islamic legal scholar Ebrahim Moosa (2003, 23),

> In terms of ethics, Muslim authorities consider the transmission of reproductive material between persons who are not legally married to be a major violation of Islamic law. This sensitivity stems from the fact that Islamic law has a strict taboo on sexual relations outside wedlock (*zina*). The taboo is designed to protect paternity (i.e., family), which is designated as one of the five goals of Islamic law, the others being the protection of religion, life, property, and reason.

As a result, at the ninth Islamic law and medicine conference, held under the auspices of the Kuwait-based Islamic Organization for Medical Sciences (IOMS) in Casablanca, Morocco, in 1997, a landmark five-point declaration included recommendations to prevent human cloning and to prohibit all situations in which a third party invades a marital relationship through donation of reproductive material (Moosa 2003). Such a ban on third-party gamete donation is effectively in place in the Sunni world, which represents approximately 80–90% of the world's 1.4 billion Muslims (Inhorn 2003, 2005; Meirow and Schenker 1997; Serour 1996, 2008; Serour and Dickens 2001).

In interviews conducted by the author with hundreds of Sunni Muslim IVF patients, they agree completely with the religious prohibitions on gamete donation, arguing that gamete donation: (1) is tantamount to adultery, by virtue of introducing a third party into the sacred dyad of husband and wife; (2) creates the potential for future half-sibling incest, if the offspring of the same anonymous donor should happen to meet and marry; and (3) confuses kinship, paternity, descent, and inheritance in the emphatically patrilineal societies of the Muslim Middle East. According to them, preserving the 'origins' of each child – meaning its relationship to a known biological mother and father – is considered not only an ideal in Islam, but a moral imperative. For Muslim men in particular, ensuring paternity and the 'purity' of lineage through 'known fathers' is of paramount concern. The problem with third-party donation, therefore, is that it destroys a child's *nasab*, or lineage, which is considered immoral in addition to being psychologically devastating. The child will be deemed illegitimate and stigmatized even in the eyes of its own parents, who will therefore lack the appropriate parental sentiments (Inhorn 2006).

This firm conviction that parenthood of a 'donor child' is an impossibility is clearly linked to the legal and cultural prohibitions against adoption throughout the Sunni Muslim world (Inhorn 1996; Sonbol 1995; Zuhur 1992). The original Al-Azhar *fatwa* prohibiting third-party gamete donation also prohibits adoption of orphans, considering both of them unallowable. As a result, few Sunni Muslim IVF patients will contemplate adopting an orphan, stating with conviction that it is 'against the religion.' According to Arab men, an adopted child, like a donor child, 'won't be my son' (Inhorn 2006).

Shia Islam and IVF

Having said this, it is very important to point out how things have changed for Shia Muslims since the beginning of the new millennium. Shia is the minority branch of Islam with its center in Iran. The countries of Iraq, Lebanon and Bahrain are thought to have Shia majorities, and Shia minority populations are also found in Syria and the eastern coast of Saudi Arabia, which is an otherwise ardently Sunni Muslim country. Shia populations can also be found in the South Asian countries of Afghanistan, Pakistan, and India, where the Ismaili and Bora Shia communities form distinct subgroups.

Many Shia religious authorities support the majority Sunni view: namely, they agree that third-party donation should be strictly prohibited. Iraq's Ayatollah Sistani, for example, has opposed any form of third-party donation (Clarke 2009). However, in the late 1990s, the Supreme Leader of the Islamic Republic of Iran, Ayatollah Ali Hussein Khamene'i, the chosen successor to Iran's Ayatollah Khomeini, issued a *fatwa* effectively permitting donor technologies to be used under certain conditions (Clarke 2006, 2009; Inhorn and Tremayne, forthcoming; Tremayne 2009). With regard to both egg and sperm donation, Ayatollah Khamene'i stated that *both* the donor and the infertile parents must abide by the religious codes regarding parenting. However, the donor child can only inherit from the sperm or egg donor, as the infertile parents are considered to be like 'adoptive' parents.

However, the situation for Shia Muslims is actually much more complicated than this. Because the Shia valorize a form of individual religious reasoning known as *ijtihad*, various Shia religious authorities have come to their own conclusions about sperm and egg donation (Mahmoud, in press; Tremayne 2009). As a result, there are now major disagreements about:

(1) whether third-party donation truly constitutes *zina*, or adultery, if no actual gaze or touch takes place with the gamete donor;

(2) whether the child should follow the name of the infertile father or the sperm donor in cases of male infertility;

(3) whether donation is permissible at all if the donors are anonymous;

(4) whether the husband of an infertile woman needs to do a temporary *mut'a* marriage with the egg donor, then release her from the marriage immediately after the embryo transfer, in order to avoid *zina*, or adultery. Such *mut'a* marriages are condoned in Shia, but condemned in Sunni Islam; and

(5) whether a Shia Muslim woman married to an infertile man can do a *mut'a* marriage with a sperm donor, which would constitute an illegal state of polyandry.

In theory, only widowed or otherwise single women – who are not currently married – should be able to accept donor sperm, in order to avoid the implications of *zina*, or adultery. However, in the Muslim countries, single motherhood of a donor child is unlikely to become socially acceptable. Indeed, Iran has disallowed sperm donation, although surrogacy has been permitted and is now widely practiced (Garmaroudi, in press). To get around this problem of sperm donation, some Iranian Shia women are temporarily divorcing their infertile husbands, temporarily marrying the sperm donors, ending the temporary marriage once the pregnancy is firmly established, and then remarrying their infertile husbands (Tremayne 2009). As Tremayne notes, such sperm donation in Iran does not necessarily make 'happy families,' suggesting the need to think through the future well-being of both women and the children conceived in this manner (Tremayne, in press).

Given these moral ambiguities and uncertainties, those married infertile Shia couples who are truly concerned about carrying out third-party donation according to religious guidelines find it difficult to meet these various requirements, particularly regarding sperm donation. Yet, having said that, in Iran and Lebanon, at least some Shia couples are beginning to receive donor gametes, as well as donating their gametes to other infertile couples. In Iranian clinics that follow Ayatollah Khamene'i's lead, all manner of egg, sperm, and embryo donation, as well as surrogacy, continue to take place, with his *fatwa* prominently displayed as moral justification (Garmaroudi, in press). Indeed, since the new millennium, donor gametes are now being donated, shared, and even purchased by infertile couples in IVF clinics in Shia-majority Iran and Lebanon, the only two countries in the Muslim world to allow this practice (Inhorn, Patrizio, and Serour, in press). For infertile Shia couples who accept the idea of donation, the introduction of donor technologies has been described as a 'marriage savior,' helping to avoid the 'marital and psychological disputes' that may arise if the couple's case is otherwise untreatable.

Who is the source of these donor gametes? In the Lebanese IVF clinics in this study, some of the donors were other IVF patients (mostly Shia Muslims who accept the idea of donation), some were friends or relatives (including egg-donor sisters), and some were anonymous donors, who provided their oocytes for a fee. In at least one clinic catering to a largely conservative Shia clientele, some of these donors were young non-Muslim, American women, who travel from the Midwest to Lebanon for extra payment in order to anonymously donate their eggs to infertile Lebanese couples. Ironically, those most likely to receive these 'American eggs' are conservative Shia couples, who accept the idea of donation because they follow the teachings of Ayatollah Khamene'i in Iran. In Lebanon, at least, such Shia recipients of American eggs are likely to be members of or sympathizers with Lebanon's Hizbullah political party, which is officially described by the US administration as a terrorist organization!

Furthermore, quite interestingly, in multi-sectarian Lebanon, the recipients of these donor eggs are not necessarily only Shia Muslim couples. Some Sunni Muslim patients from Lebanon and from other Middle Eastern Muslim countries such as Egypt and Syria are quietly slipping across transnational borders to 'save their marriages' through the use of donor gametes, thereby secretly 'going against' the dictates of Sunni Muslim orthodoxy. That such reproductive travel is done in secrecy – usually under the guise of a 'holiday in Beirut' – is quite important, given the moral condemnation of gamete donation in the Sunni Muslim countries. Although such Sunni Muslim gamete seekers may have made peace with their own moral decisions to use donor technologies, they often remain extremely concerned about maintaining anonymity and confidentiality, in order to avoid moral censure of themselves and their future donor offspring. The story of Hatem and Huda, a long-term infertile Muslim couple, bespeaks the complexities within the Middle Eastern reproscape.

The story of Hatem and Huda's secret egg quest

Hatem and Huda were patients in a hospital-based IVF clinic in Beirut that catered to all of the religious sects found in multi-sectarian Lebanon. However, Hatem and Huda were not Lebanese, having traveled from rural Syria to Beirut in order to undergo a cycle of IVF. Like most Syrian reproductive tourists, Hatem was convinced that Lebanese IVF clinics were superior to the fledgling clinics in neighboring Syria, a Middle Eastern nation-state that has long been isolated from, and even sanctioned by, the West. Thus, he had been bringing his wife to Beirut for IVF since 1997. Hatem had another reason for bringing Huda to Lebanon: there, they could access donor eggs, which were unavailable in the Sunni-dominant country of Syria, where third-party gamete donation is strictly prohibited.

First cousins married for 17 years, Hatem and Huda clearly loved each other, despite the perplexing dilemma of her premature ovarian failure. Although Huda was only 36 at the time, she had entered menopause in her 20s, and required hormonal stimulation followed by IVF in order to achieve a pregnancy. After five unsuccessful trials of IVF, the IVF physicians in Beirut recommended egg donation as the most likely successful option. As Sunni Muslims, Hatem and Huda knew that egg donation was forbidden in the religion. Yet, as Hatem explained, they rationalized their use of donor eggs in a previous IVF cycle in the following way,

> As long as the donor agrees, then this would reduce the *haram* [forbiddenness] based on our religion. Because she, the donor, is in need of money, she gave nine to ten eggs, and the doctor divided the eggs between that couple and us. We took five, and that couple,

who were recently married, took five. And I personally entered into the lab to make sure that *my* sperm were being used. It's okay because it's *my* sperm.

Indeed, Huda became pregnant with donor twins, a male and a female, in 1999. At six months and 17 days of pregnancy, she began to miscarry, and Hatem rushed her to a hospital in Syria. As Hatem recounts,

> They opened her stomach [by cesarean], and there were twins, who still lived for 48 hours. They had lung deficiency because they were little and not fully developed. The girl died twelve hours before the boy.

After this traumatic experience, Huda could no longer accept the idea of egg donation. According to Hatem, who spoke for Huda as she sat quietly in the room,

> She was tortured [during the pregnancy]. She stayed four months vomiting whatever she ate, and she lost weight – from 88 kilograms to 55 kilograms. And she was under a lot of stress because of our social environment in Syria. In our [farming] community, they stare at babies and see if they resemble the mother and father. We are not living in a city of 4–5 million. We are in a closed community of 15,000 people. And so, the first time, when we had twins, they did a blood test and everyone was surprised. Their blood group was AB, and it didn't match ours. Now everyone will *really* examine the personal traits of this [donor] baby if we do it again. They will look at us suspiciously. Not the doctors; they keep everything confidential. But people in the community who might come to visit and look at us curiously.

For his part, Hatem is willing to accept donor eggs again and has already made inquiries about finding a willing Shia Muslim egg donor in Syria. On the day of his interview, he also spoke about the possibility of finding a willing donor within the Beirut IVF clinic. Hatem saw no other way to achieve parenthood, given that he loves his wife and refuses to divorce her. Although Hatem is an affluent farmer from a large family of 20 children (by one father and three co-wives), he continues to resist all forms of social pressure to divorce or marry polygynously. His commitment, he says, is based on his deep love for Huda. As he said,

> Had I not loved her, I wouldn't have waited for seventeen years. I would have married another. By religious law, I can remarry, but I don't want to. She told me I should marry another woman, and she even offered or suggested that she would get me engaged, because we're already old. We've reached middle age without kids. We're living in a large family with six of my brothers, and they all have children. That's why she's feeling very depressed and very angry that she's alone without children, although she's always surrounded by children. But, of course, she keeps these feelings to herself.
>
> The love between us – I love her *a lot*. I was the one who considered going for IVF, for her sake. But we must keep it secret, because if my parents knew about us having an IVF child, the child would be marginalized and living a lonely life. So we keep everything secret, and we just mention to our families that she's receiving treatment.

As in so many IVF stories, Huda and Hatem were ultimately unsuccessful in their seventh attempted IVF cycle. Huda's own eggs failed to mature under hormonal stimulation, and no egg donors were currently available at the clinic. Thus, Hatem and Huda returned home quietly to Syria, with little remaining hope of achieving parenthood, but with the love that had kept them together for nearly twenty years.

Conclusion

The arrival of donor technologies in both Lebanon and Iran – the only two Middle Eastern countries to offer these services at the present time – has led to a brave new world of reproductive possibility never imagined when ARTs were first introduced there exactly 25 years ago. These technologies have engendered significant medical transnationalism and reproductive tourism; mixing of gametes across national, ethnic, racial, and religious lines; and the birth of thousands of donor babies to devout infertile Muslim couples. For their part, at least some infertile Muslim couples, both Shia and Sunni, have begun to reconsider traditional notions of *nasab*, or the meaning of biological lineage, even if 'social parenthood' of a donor child is still not widely embraced in the Middle Eastern Muslim world (Inhorn 2006). Nonetheless, because donor technologies are now widely available in both Iran and Lebanon, the power of the Sunni Muslim ban on third-party donation is being weakened across the region, with some infertile Sunni Muslim couples such as Hatem and Huda reconsidering their own anti-donation moral stances. As a result of these social processes, Shia gametes are finding their ways into Sunni bodies, despite the current regional tensions and sometimes outright antagonisms between these branches of Islam. Indeed, in the new millennium, hundreds – perhaps even thousands – of infertile Sunni Muslim couples are traveling abroad in search of such Shia donor gametes.

As suggested by the Middle Eastern reproscape, reproductive travel is a growing global phenomenon (Blyth and Farrand 2005; Deech 2003; Pennings 2002), one that needs to be studied by medical anthropologists. Anthropologists are exceptionally well positioned to gather important ethnographic information from reproductive travelers themselves, thereby understanding the motivations that compel them to seek ARTs outside their own countries. In doing so, our discipline can serve to humanize the legal and policy discourses on this subject, and to shed light on both the macro-and micro-level dynamics of the global reproscape, which is still shrouded in mystery.

The author's own multi-sited ethnographic investigation of the Middle Eastern reproscape has begun to uncover the motivations of a diverse set of infertile men and women as they travel to and from ART sites within the region and beyond. Indeed, global travel is part and parcel of the modern-day quest for conception among Middle Eastern Muslim couples. The deployment of the most high-tech forms of assisted reproduction is a facet of Middle Eastern modernity that is rarely emphasized in either the sparse literature on Islamic technoscience (Lotfalian 2004), or in Western polemics on the 'backwardness' of the region (see also Deeb 2006). Moreover, such modernity is being supported by Islamic juridical and bioethical discourses, which are being used to justify various forms of technological assistance, while limiting others (Inhorn and Tremayne, in press). Islamic bioethics have caught the attention of a new generation of Middle Eastern Studies scholars, who in recent years, have compiled four edited volumes on this subject (Brockopp 2003; Brockopp and Eich 2008; Hamid and Grewal 2011; Inhorn and Tremayne, in press). In short, although the Middle East is rarely regarded in this way, it is a key site for understanding the intersection of technoscience, religious morality, and modernity, all of which are deeply implicated in the Middle Eastern reproscape.

Acknowledgements

The author wishes to thank Harish Naraindas and Cristiana Bastos for inviting her into this special issue. She is also extremely grateful to two particularly perceptive and creative reviewers, who engaged seriously with this paper, its wish for a new and better vocabulary to describe reproductive 'tourism,' and its exploration of Islamic discourses on ARTs. One reviewer provided particularly helpful feedback on the expansion of Arjun Appadurai's work. The other provided useful cautionary advice to avoid essentializing Islam and its Sunni and Shia variants, as well as the notion of romantic love. The author has attempted to answer most of the reviewers' suggestions, and has referenced a new and growing body of work on Islamic bioethics and Islam and ARTs, which deals with many of the nuances beyond those contained in this brief article. Mostly, the author thanks the many gracious and candid women and men who have participated in her ethnographic research on infertility and ARTs in the Middle East. This research was approved by the Behavioral Science Institutional Review Boards (IRB) at the University of Michigan and Yale University's Human Subjects Committee (HSC). Final thanks go to the US Department of Education Fulbright-Hays Faculty Research Abroad Program and the National Science Foundation's Cultural Anthropology Program for generous funding of this research. No conflicts of interest occurred.

Notes

1. This article is based on long-term ethnographic fieldwork conducted in multiple Middle Eastern countries, including Egypt, Lebanon, United Arab Emirates, Iran, and 'Arab Detroit,' and representing nearly 600 Middle Eastern couples (primarily from Egypt, Lebanon, Syria, Palestine, the United Arab Emirates, Iraq, and Yemen). This article is based primarily on the author's two most recent studies, one on male infertility carried out in Beirut, Lebanon in 2003, and the other on reproductive tourism carried out in the United Arab Emirates in 2007. In addition, fieldwork among infertile Arab Americans took place from 2003–2005 and 2007–2008.
2. The term 'bioscope' is the author's own, but bespeaks the strong Foucauldian influences in medical anthropology, where terms such as 'biopower,' 'biopolitics,' 'biocitizenship,' 'bioavailability,' and 'biocrossings' are becoming common parlance.
3. Thanks to one of the reviewers for suggesting this composite term.

References

Appadurai, Arjun. 1990. Disjuncture and difference in the global cultural economy. In *Global culture: Nationalism, globalization and identity*, ed. Mike Featherstone, 296–308. London: Sage.

Appadurai, Arjun. 1996. *Modernity at large: Cultural dimensions of globalization*. Minneapolis: University of Minnesota Press.

Basch, Linda, Nina Glick Schiller, and Cristina Szanton Blanc. 1994. *Nations unbound: Transnational projects, postcolonial predicaments, and deterritorialized nation-states*. Langhorne, PA: Gordon and Breach.

Blank, Robert. 1998. Regulation of donor insemination. In *Donor insemination: International social science perspectives*, ed. Ken Daniels and Erica Haimes, 131–150. Cambridge, UK: Cambridge University Press.

Blyth, Eric, and Abigail Farrand. 2005. Reproductive tourism – a price worth paying for reproductive autonomy? *Critical Social Policy* 25: 91–114.

Blyth, Eric, and Ruth Landau, eds. 2004. *Third party assisted conception across cultures: Social, legal and ethical perspectives*. London: Jessica Kingsley.

Braverman, Andrea M. 2001. Exploring ovum donors' motivations and needs. *The American Journal of Bioethics* 1: 16–17.

Brockopp, Jonathan E., ed. 2003. *Islamic ethics of life: Abortion, war, and euthanasia*. Columbia: University of South Carolina Press.

Brockopp, Jonathan E., and Thomas Eich, eds. 2008. *Muslim medical ethics: From theory to practice*. Columbia: University of South Carolina Press.

Carmeli, Yoram S., and Daphna Birenbaum-Carmeli. 2000. Ritualizing the 'natural family': secrecy in Israeli donor insemination. *Science as Culture* 9: 301–24.

Clarke, Morgan. 2006. Shiite perspectives on kinship and new reproductive technologies. *ISIM Newsletter* 17: 26–7.

Clarke, Morgan. 2009. *Islam and new kinship: Reproductive technology and the Shariah in Lebanon.* New York: Berghahn Books.

Cohen, Lawrence. 1999. Where it hurts: Indian material for an ethics of organ transplantation. *Daedalus* 128: 135–64.

Cohen, Lawrence. 2002. The other kidney: Biopolitics beyond recognition. In *Commodifying Bodies,* ed. Nancy Scheper-Hughes and Loic Wacquant, 9–29. London: Sage.

Deeb, Lara. 2006. *An enchanted modern: Gender and public piety in Shi'i Lebanon.* Princeton, NJ: Princeton University Press.

Deech, Ruth. 2003. Reproductive tourism in Europe: Infertility and human rights. *Global Governance* 9: 425–32.

Franklin, Sarah. 1996. *Embodied progress: A cultural account of assisted conception.* London: Routledge.

Friedman, Jonathan. 1994. *Cultural identity and global process.* London: Sage.

Garmaroudi, Shirin Naef. Forthcoming. Gestational surrogacy in Iran; Uterine kinship and the notion of reproduction in Shia thought and practice. In *Islam and assisted reproductive technologies: Sunni and Shia perspectives,* ed. Marcia C. Inhorn and Soraya Tremayne. New York: Berghahn Books.

Ginsburg, Faye D., and Rayna Rapp. 1995. Introduction: Conceiving the new world order. In *Conceiving the new world order: The global politics of reproduction,* ed. Faye D. Ginsburg and Rayna Rapp, 1–17. Berkeley: University of California Press.

Hamid, Hamada, and Zareena Grewal. 2011. *Treating muslims.* Thousand Oaks, CA: Sage.

Hannerz, Ulf. 1996. *Transnational connections: Culture, people, places.* London: Routledge.

Heng, BC. 2007. Regulatory safeguards needed for the travelling foreign egg donor. *Human Reproduction* 22: 2350–2.

Inhorn, Marcia C. 1994. *Quest for conception: Gender, infertility, and Egyptian medical traditions.* Philadelphia: University of Pennsylvania Press.

Inhorn, Marcia C. 1996. *Infertility and patriarchy: The cultural politics of gender and family life in Egypt.* Philadelphia: University of Pennsylvania Press.

Inhorn, Marcia C. 2003. *Local babies, global science: Gender, religion, and in vitro fertilization in Egypt.* New York: Routledge.

Inhorn, Marcia C. 2005. *Fatwas* and ARTs: IVF and gamete donation in Sunni v. Shi'a Islam. *Journal of Gender, Race & Justice* 9: 291–317.

Inhorn, Marcia C. 2006. 'He won't be my son': Middle Eastern Muslim men's discourses of adoption and gamete donation. *Medical Anthropology Quarterly* 20: 94–120.

Inhorn, Marcia C. 2007. Loving your infertile Muslim spouse: Notes on the globalization of IVF and its romantic commitments in Sunni Egypt and Shi'ite Lebanon. In *Love and globalization: Transformations of intimacy in the contemporary world,* eds. Mark B. Padilla, Jennifer S. Hirsch, Miguel Munoz-Laboy, Robert Sember, and Richard G. Parker, 139–160. Nashville, TN: Vanderbilt University Press.

Inhorn, Marcia C. 2009. Right to assisted reproductive technology: Overcoming infertility in low-resource countries. *International Journal of Gynecology and Obstetrics* 106: 172–4.

Inhorn, Marcia C., and Pasquale Patrizio. 2009. Rethinking reproductive 'tourism' as reproductive 'exile'. *Fertility and Sterility* 92: 904–6.

Inhorn, Marcia C., and Pankaj Shrivistav. 2010. Globalization and reproductive tourism in the United Arab Emirates. *Asia-Pacific Journal of Public Health* 22 (Suppl): 68–74.

Inhorn, Marcia C., and Soraya Tremayne, eds. Forthcoming. *Islam and assisted reproductive technologies: Sunni and Shia perspectives.* New York: Berghahn Press.

Inhorn, Marcia C., Pasquale Patrizio, and Gamal I. Serour. Forthcoming. Third-party reproductive assistance around the Mediterranean: Comparing Sunni Egypt, Catholic

Italy, and multi-sectarian Lebanon. In *Islam and assisted reproductive technologies: Sunni and Shia perspectives*, ed. Marcia C. Inhorn and Soraya Tremayne. New York: Berghahn Books.

Kahn, Susan Martha. 2000. *Reproducing Jews: A cultural account of assisted conception in Israel*. Durham, NC: Duke University Press.

Kirkman, Maggie. 2003. Egg and embryo donation and the meaning of motherhood. *Women & Health* 38: 1–18.

Kleinman, Arthur. 1995. *Writing at the margin: Discourse between anthropology and medicine*. Berkeley: University of California Press.

Konrad, Monica. 1998. Ova donation and symbols of substance: Some variations on the theme of sex, gender and the partible body. *The Journal of the Royal Anthropological Institute* 4: 643–67.

Lee, Felicia R. 2005. Fertility tourists go great lengths to conceive. *The New York Times*, January 25.

Lewellen, Ted C. 2002. *The anthropology of globalization: Cultural anthropology enters the 21st century*. Westport, CT: Bergin and Garvey.

Lock, Margaret. 2001. *Twice dead: Organ transplants and the reinvention of death*. Berkeley: University of California Press.

Lorber, Judith. 1989. Choice, gift, or patriarchal bargain? Women's consent to *in vitro* fertilization in male infertility. *Hypatia* 4: 23–36.

Lotfalian, Mazyar. 2004. *Islam, technoscientific identities, and the culture of curiosity*. Dallas: University Press of America.

Mahmoud, Farouk. Forthcoming. Controversies in Islamic evaluation of assisted reproductive technologies. In *Islam and assisted reproductive technologies: Sunni and Shia perspectives*, ed. Marcia C. Inhorn and Soraya Tremayne. New York: Berghahn Books.

Meirow, D., and J.G. Schenker. 1997. The current status of sperm donation in assisted reproduction technology: Ethical and legal considerations. *Journal of Assisted Reproduction and Genetics* 14: 133–8.

Moosa, Ebrahim. 2003. Human cloning in Muslim ethics. *Voices Across Boundaries* Fall: 23–26.

Musallam, B.F. 1986. *Sex and society in Islam: Birth control before the nineteenth century*. Cambridge, UK: Cambridge University Press.

Ong, Aihwa, and Stephen J. Collier, eds. 2005. *Global assemblages: Technology, politics, and ethics as anthropological problems*. Malden, MA: Blackwell.

Pennings, G. 2002. Reproductive tourism as moral pluralism in motion. *Journal of Medical Ethics* 28: 337–41.

Pollock, Anne. 2003. Complicating power in high-tech reproduction: Narratives of anonymous paid egg donors. *Journal of Medical Humanities* 24: 241–63.

Ritzer, George, ed. 2002. *McDonaldization: The reader*. Thousand Oaks, CA: Pine Forge Press.

Schaebler, Birgit, and Leif Stenberg. 2004. *Globalization and the Muslim world: Culture, religion, and modernity*. Syracuse, NY: Syracuse University Press.

Scheper-Hughes, Nancy. 2000. The global traffic in human organs. *Current Anthropology* 41: 191–211.

Scheper-Hughes, Nancy. 2002a. Bodies for sale – whole or in parts. In *Commodifying bodies*, ed. Nancy Scheper-Hughes and Loic Wacquant, 1–8. London: Sage.

Scheper-Hughes, Nancy. 2002b. The ends of the body: Commodity fetishism and the global traffic in organs. *SAIS Review* 23: 61–80.

Serour, Gamal I. 1996. Bioethics in reproductive health: A Muslim's perspective. *Middle East Fertility Society Journal* 1: 30–5.

Serour, Gamal. I. 2008. Islamic perspectives in human reproduction. *Reproductive BioMedicine Online* 17, Suppl. 3: 34–8.

Serour, G.I., and B.M. Dickens. 2001. Assisted reproduction developments in the Islamic world. *International Journal of Gynecology & Obstetrics* 74: 187–93.

Shanley, Mary Lyndon. 2002. Collaboration and commodification in assisted procreation: Reflections on an open market and anonymous donation in human sperm and eggs. *Law & Society Review* 36: 257–83.

Sharp, Lesley A. 2000. The commodification of the body and its parts. *Annual Review of Anthropology* 29: 287–328.

Sharp, Lesley A. 2006. *Strange harvest: Organ transplants, denatured bodies, and the transformed self.* Berkeley: University of California Press.

Sonbol, Amira el Azhary. 1995. Adoption in Islamic society: A historical survey. In *Children in the Muslim Middle East*, ed. Fernea Elizabeth Warnock. Austin: University of Texas Press.

Spar, Debora. 2005. Reproductive tourism and the regulatory map. *The New England Journal of Medicine* 352: 531–3.

Storrow, Richard F. 2005. Quests for conception: Fertility tourists, globalization, and feminist legal theory. *Hastings Law Journal* 57: 295–330.

Thompson, Charis M. 2005. *Making parents: The ontological choreography of reproductive technologies.* Cambridge, MA: MIT Press.

Tremayne, Soraya. 2009. Law, ethics, and donor technologies in Shia Iran. In *Assisting reproduction, testing genes: Global encounters with new biotechnologies*, ed. Daphna Birenbaum-Carmeli and Marcia C. Inhorn, 144–63. New York: Berghahn Books.

Van der Ploeg, Irma. 1995. Hermaphrodite patients: In vitro fertilization and the transformation of male infertility. *Science, Technology, & Human Values* 460–81.

Zuhur, Sherifa, 1992. Of milk-mothers and sacred bonds: Islam, patriarchy, and new reproductive technologies. *Creighton Law Review* 25: 1725–38.

Affective journeys: the emotional structuring of medical tourism in India

Harris Solomon

Department of Anthropology, Brown University, Providence, RI, USA

This paper examines the grid of sentiment that structures medical travel to India. In contrast to studies that render emotion as ancillary, the paper argues that affect is fundamental to medical travel's ability to ease the linked somatic, emotional, financial, and political injuries of being ill 'back home'. The ethnographic approach follows the scenes of medical travel within the Indian corporate hospital room, based on observations and interviews among foreign patients, caregivers, and hospital staff in Mumbai, New Delhi, Chennai, and Bangalore. Foreign patients conveyed diverse sentiments about their journey to India ranging from betrayal to gratitude, and their expressions of risk, healthcare costs, and cultural difference help sustain India's popularity as a medical travel destination. However, although the affective dimensions of medical travel promise a remedy for foreign patients, they also reveal the fault lines of market medicine in India.

On December 9, 2009, the American television commentator Glenn Beck threaded his signature angry sarcasm through a report on labour union politics. Explaining how the Service Employees International Union (SEIU) was 'reciprocating' with President Obama for his support, Beck noted that the SEIU's website 'is promoting the greatness of the health care system in India'. He screened a video clip from the SEIU webpage of an American woman who travelled to New Delhi for a hip replacement that cost her $12,500, and who questioned the $50,000 price tag for the same procedure in the US. Beck turned to the camera and said plainly, 'The best I can figure is all that money goes to high-tech hospitals and doctors who studied at Harvard rather than Gajra Raja Medical School... if you have a choice between getting hip replacement surgery at the Mumbai clinic at Punjab, or the Mayo Clinic, I'm going to go for the Mayo clinic' (Beck 2009; Haniffa 2009). Although he did not term it as such, Beck was ridiculing the phenomenon of 'medical tourism', whereby patients travel to a different country for their healthcare to circumvent high costs, Gordian insurance policies and lengthy treatment wait-times. Among many destination countries, such as Mexico, Thailand, Costa Rica, and Brazil, increasingly such patients are choosing to travel to India for their medical care.[1]

Although Beck's disdainful framing of medical travel precluded the possibility that India (a place whose holy river Ganges, he remarked, 'sounds like a disease') could provide high-quality medical care to Americans, a different narrative is unfolding in India's 'super-specialty' marble and glass corporate hospitals. In one such hospital, set off a Bangalore highway and emblazoned with an Ivy League university shield on its exterior, this author sat with the head of international patient services, Mr Krishnan.[2] Mr Krishnan noted that his staff are specially trained to take care of American and British patients, and that the hospital's affiliation with an esteemed US university gives confidence to foreign patients. 'India has positioned itself as tertiary care for the outside world,' he said, more than any other country. 'People trust us with their lives, because caring is part of the Indian tradition.'

Medical tourism makes health a comparative enterprise, wherein treatment options go beyond second opinions and stretch to second countries. Entangled within this journey of comparative consumer choice is an intensely affective reckoning with deep forms of difference. In India, medical tourism's critics have described how it ironically shifts India's place in the colonial medical imaginary, such that 'in spite of fundamental policy failures in public health, India is increasingly seen as an attractive international healthcare destination (Ananthakrishnan 2006). The underbelly of this attraction has even surfaced in popular fiction. For example, Robin Cook's medical thriller *Foreign Body* tells the story of an American medical student who embarks on a quest to India to solve a series of unexplained deaths of elderly Americans who travelled there for low-cost surgery (Cook 2008). These parables of curative exotics and racialized suspicions channel powerful public sentiment, from Beck's insults to the horror of Cook's novel, and from frustrations with roadblocks to healing to the happiness of satisfied patients returned from India.

This paper examines the grid of sentiment that structures the relations between nations, bodies, and forms of care produced through medical travel to India. On these affective journeys, medical travel to India eases linked somatic, emotional, financial, and political injuries of being ill 'back home'. Medical tourism's advocates in India and many foreign patients frame healthcare in the West as inconvenient, expensive, and often hopeless, and assert that India is a place to repair possibilities for hope and healing. Some Indian doctors engage medical tourism as a form of postcolonial critique, and contend that its popularity marks a repair to the imbalance of medical modernity, whereby the hubris of the West has left its citizens sick and stranded, only to be rescued by India's technological ascent. In this circumstance, affect intensifies relations between patients, caregivers, and spaces of care both distant and immediate. The paper's ethnographic focus follows the scenes of medical travel that unfold within the Indian corporate hospital room, a space that materializes the array of sentiments generated through patients' journeys.

The paper's perspective on affect builds on an extensive literature in anthropology and the social sciences concerned with emotions and the structure of caregiving (Lutz 1986; Hochschild 2003). This scholarship does not counter emotion against rationality, or nature against culture; by contrast, it takes seemingly contradictory stances as cultural forms unto themselves (Lutz and White 1986) and as constitutive elements of contemporary public culture (Mazzarella 2009). Affective atmospheres also connect to orders of power and resources that both enable and withhold care, reflected in Sara Ahmed's term 'affective economy' and in Ann Stoler's notion of 'emotional economy' that specifies 'when, where, and with whom sentiments were withheld, demanded, and 'freely' displayed' (Ahmed 2004; Stoler 2002, 168).[3] Both poetic and political, these contingencies are 'available to be worked upon through a whole series of new entities and institutions' exemplified by the assemblage of transnational medical travel (Thrift 2007, 192).

To date, ethnographic engagements with medical travel have focused on the intentions of patients to travel, the problems posed for local communities in 'destination' countries, or prescriptions for future anthropological studies (Augé 1985; Gray and Poland 2008; Kangas 2002, 2007; Sobo 2009; Song 2010; Whittaker 2008, 2009), and a select few engage the issue in India (Bhardwaj 2008; Kangas 2007). These studies clarify medical travel's circuits of bodies and technologies, and begin to address Sobo's (2009) call for anthropologists to disentangle medical tourism's oversimplification as 'globalisation' by many popular media sources. However, although these studies often acknowledge the hope, anxiety, and anger generated through medical travel, some tend to render emotion as ancillary.

By contrast, this paper argues that affect is fundamental to and constitutive of medical travel. Following Biehl, Coutinho, and Outeiro (2001, 94), it considers the affective dimensions of medical travel as 'the new material and medium through which contemporary technoscientific mechanisms of governance are made up' (also see Adams, Murphy, and Clarke 2009; Iedema, Jorm, and Lum 2009; Patel 2007). Thinking about medical travel in this way helps illuminate its mechanics of scale, whereby affect is the linchpin between everyday sentiments and objects, clinical care, and medical travel's institutional structuring. For example, the affect of anticipation guides the journeys of patients seeking what they could not find at home, but it also conditions the handshakes among hospital and government officials that ultimately deem foreigners as possessing more 'return' on investments in healthcare (Adams, Murphy, and Clarke 2009). The affective moments of medical travel mediate locations and scales, from hospital rooms to Ministries of Health to insurance agencies. 'Mediate' is used intentionally here to point to the active force of affect, following Latour's (2005, 39) definition of 'mediators' as forces that 'transform, translate, distort, and modify the meaning or the elements they are supposed to carry'.

Drawing medical travel into these analytics, then, connects transnational forms of biomedical capital (Sunder Rajan 2006) to powerful instances of what Kathleen Stewart terms 'ordinary affects' (Stewart 2007). According to Stewart, everyday forms of emotion, relation, and recognition 'highlight the question of the intimate impact of forces in circulation. They're not exactly "personal" but they sure can pull the subject into places it didn't exactly "intend" to go' (Stewart 2007, 40). The sentiments instantiated through medical tourism exemplify this pull and push of subjects: across geographic borders, through healthcare's apparent dead-ends of solemn resignation and promising, unexpected detours, and into relations with caregivers far from home. On these paths, affect mediates medical travel by connecting illness to consumer choice, and a perceived failure of home healthcare systems to hopes about circumventing them in India. Ordinary affects are not bystanders in life, according to Stewart; instead they give life form. To avoid taking the circuits and flows of medical travel for granted, the paper focuses specifically on the moments of affect that mediate them.

However fragmented and mobile, though, these moments cohere in discrete spaces. Navaro-Yashin (2009) focuses on this process of spatialization, by questioning the extent to which recent ethnographies deem affect a matter of interior subjectivity versus a matter of interactions between humans, objects, and environments.[4]

Reflecting on her field research in Northern Cyprus, Navaro-Yashin uses the term 'affective spaces' to bridge the mutual influences of subject, object, and environment. She writes that her informants' subjectivities 'were shaped by and embroiled in the ruins which surrounded them,' but 'the affect of the ruins had a subjective quality, too' (Navaro-Yashin 2009, 15). Similarly, the hospital room operates as a relational, transformational space for medical travel. It bears witness to and conditions a journey focused on India which is constantly in relation to prior injuries back home.

Comparative values

Patterns of foreigners travelling to India for medical care have an extensive history that predates their more recent publicity, due to services and/or technologies unavailable in the patient's place of origin (Kangas 2002) and to historically contingent ideas about illness and geography (Roberts, forthcoming). The destinations for this travel often are corporate hospitals owned by Indian companies that grew during the 1990s' market liberalisation within a landscape of tiered public-private healthcare facilities in Indian metros (Baru 2005; Duggal 1996; Lefebvre 2008).[5] Along with advanced technology, these facilities offer a sense of care and empathy that Indians across socio-economic divides complain is missing from overburdened and understaffed government facilities. The affect of care advertised to foreigners is one cultivated in high-end hospitals and reserved for anyone, whether Indian or foreign, who is willing to pay for it.[6] Tie-ups between hospitals and American, European, and Indian 'virtual broker' medical travel companies help arrange procedures for international patients based on the premise of quality at low cost.

Two distinct but linked origin stories account for medical tourism's recent growth in India, which is estimated to yield 100 billion rupees (US$2.3 billion) by 2012, according to a consultancy report by McKinsey and Company (Confederation of Indian Industry 2002).[7] One credits the 'IT boom' that brought India international visibility for its technical acumen, and the other credits the Indian-owned Icon Hospital with the marketing know-how and mastery of giving medical tourism its appealing spin. Indian health rights advocates are quick to point out, however, that medical tourism is not exactly a private venture, because it enjoys 'soft' forms of support from the Indian government, including tariff reductions for expensive equipment, discounts on land prices to hospitals, and regulatory oversight that allows the hospitals to shirk their obligations of a minimum amount of indigent care that is the precondition for government support. Such public-sector support for medical tourism, its critics argue, deflects attention and resources away from the public healthcare sector (Ananthakrishnan 2006; Sengupta 2008; Sengupta and Nundy 2005). The Government of India's visible involvement includes a 2002 National Health Policy that explicitly encourages medical tourism, a system of medical tourism councils set up at the state level, and a new visa category for foreign patients and their accompanying caregivers (Government of India 2002; Ananthakrishnan 2006).

The data for this paper come from six months of observations and interviews during 2005 and 2006, consisting of observations of patient and caregiver interactions; 30 open-ended interviews with patients and doctors in several corporate, NGO, and government hospitals, clinics, and research centres; and 15 interviews with staff in healthcare-related public relations offices and media agencies in Mumbai, New Delhi, Chennai, and Bangalore. The clinical contexts varied widely, as the destinations for medical tourism range from corporate hospitals to 'trust' hospitals set up by charities or other non-governmental organisations. Others, although far less often the case, are government, public sector hospitals.[8] This paper concentrates on one particular corporate hospital, called 'Icon Hospital', whose branches the author visited in several cities, and whose patients from the US and Europe were interviewed along with medical staff.[9] Icon's extensive involvement in medical tourism prompted the choice to focus on its hospitals as primary ethnographic sites.

British and American patients are the focus here because the author is American and was most often introduced to (non-Indian) American or British patients by hospital staff who were ever-present gatekeepers during this research. Left aside, reluctantly, are the narratives of non-resident Indian (NRI) patients, and of patients from South Asia, the Middle East, and Africa, such as Iraqis seeking advanced wound care and Tanzanian parents who received support from a charity to bring their infant to India for heart surgery. Often, waiting room observations entailed conversations with Indian patients who were travellers themselves, coming from smaller towns or rural areas to the metropoles for treatment. For example, in a waiting room in Chennai, an auto repairman from central India waited for his aunt to come out of daylong diagnostic tests for her unexplained joint pain. He explained in Hindi that they did not want to go to a 'branch' – a smaller hospital – but rather a flagship facility, despite the distance from home. As Inhorn and Patrizio (2009) suggest in their concept of 'reproductive exile', a sense of forced relocation sets the limits of 'choice' in medical travel, which remains a reality for many Indians who navigate uneven opportunities for care yet whose experiences rarely if ever filter through medical tourism's broader discursive formation.

The multi-sited ethnographic approach described here enabled a comparative inquiry across regions of India and across clinical contexts, but it also limited patient visits and follow-up, meaning that the analysis ends at discharge and therefore remains speculative regarding 'the journey' beyond the hospital visit. Indian friends often joked that the project was focused on five-star hotels, as they called corporate hospitals, spaces that Lawrence Cohen (1995, 327) describes as 'hermetically sealed, creating through air conditioning and subdued colour schemes an anti-tropical space'. This isolation means that for many foreign patients, their experience of India unfolds principally in the hospital, and their interactions with Indians are limited largely to medical professionals. This also holds true for the ethnographer engaged with them: 'the field' is separated sharply from the quotidian bustle of an Indian urban centre, within institutions that take pride in carefully calibrating how India appears in their halls and encounters. A sense of the generic infuses these interiors, yet despite the hospital room's globalized, English-speaking, biomedical frame, patients (and the researcher) felt compelled to reconcile it with the vernacular. The paper describes these attempts at connection through the narratives of two foreign patients at Icon, one from the US and one from the UK. Materialized sometimes in the briefest of encounters, their affective journeys reveal the intimate textures of healthcare across geographic bounds.

Rubles and rupees

Walking through the international patient ward of Icon Hospital, Gautham, who worked in Icon's international patient services unit, explained that the hospital sponsors training sessions for its staff in 'cultural awareness' as it relates to national preference, and shared mnemonics he learned such as 'Americans need personal space' and 'the British enjoy silence'. In the quiet, sleek ward, he made introductions to Bill and Judy Jackson, a couple in their 50s hailing from a town near a southern stretch of Interstate 95. Bill was propped up on his hospital bed, and Judy sat cross-legged on the sofa next to him in a pink warm-up suit. Bill was soon to go in for orthopaedic surgery after several days of pre-op tests. Bill and Judy were in India because they are two of nearly 46 million non-elderly uninsured Americans (Henry J. Kaiser Family Foundation 2008). By coming to India, they planned to save at least $100,000 in medical costs associated with a surgery deemed immediately necessary by Bill's doctors in the US, but whose American price tag was out of their reach.[10] When Bill's doctors suggested that he explore the option of coming to India, Judy searched online and discovered Globe Health, one of a growing number of 'virtual brokers' of medical tourism, and began exchanging emails with their representative. The calculus of cost quickly became self-evident, and guided by the staff of Globe Health, Judy began the process of working towards a trip to India: getting immunisations, corralling Bill's medical records, submitting passport applications, making airline reservations, and establishing a line of communication with Gautham's office at Icon. Globe Health facilitated several of these elements, from travel arrangements to in-country administrative details. Judy and Bill paid Globe Health a fee in exchange for these 'concierge' services.[11]

Judy thought the staff in the hospital were kind, and that they take better care of a patient than in the US. But these advantages, she said, had to be put alongside the challenges of their first visit to India, including their responses to crowds, poverty, and a different set of sense stimuli: 'Some of the smells are really horrific, and it's hard to get past the smell to eat... I don't mind trying different things... it's just Indian food... the smell.' These criticisms were each prefaced by an apology to Gautham, who stood by Bill's bed and responded with a polite nod of acknowledgment. Gautham assured them that these issues were commonplace for Western visitors and that Icon prides itself in being able to offer specially catered meals.

Bill said that their confidence came in part from Indian friends back home who highly recommended Icon Hospital, and this helped ease an abiding sense of fear they had of coming to India: 'We're just some Southern people, we've never been outside the United States, and we were kinda scared stark.' The Jacksons came with their two college-age children, who were staying in a local hotel and exploring the city. Bill explained that their kids hired a taxi to travel around, and noted that it cost 'eleven hundred rubles, whatever that is,' and turned to Gautham to ask: 'How much is that in American money?' Gautham immediately replied, 'I'll have to check the exchange rate, sir – we don't have any rubles.' This added to the mix-up, and prompted Bill to ask, 'Well, what's ya'll's money called here?' Gautham responded, 'Rupees, sir, rupees.' Bill's confusion about currency was perfectly understandable: although he had been in India for a week, he hadn't seen or touched Indian money. The currency of their experience was dollars saved as much as it was rupees spent. He and Judy were taken directly from the airport to the hospital in a car provided by Icon as part of their package deal on Bill's surgery. They had not and likely would not leave the hospital during their estimated 5-week stay, until it came time for their return home.

The 'cashless experience' of Bill's procedure is central to advertisements about medical tourism to India. It evokes a hospital stay that is painless, worry-free, and door-to-door smooth, although Bill and Judy's uneasiness, worked out in nervous laughter with Gautham, belied this promise. It also is foundational to what Gautham described as Icon's plans for tie-ups with American insurance companies so that 'all you have to do is produce your card, whoever is your life or health insurance person. With your number, we'll process it.'[12] The Jacksons would be swiping a different card – their credit card – making the trade-off of travelling to India in order to ease their healthcare debt. Gautham emphasized that Bill's experience at Icon was shaping him to become a 'brand ambassador' upon his return to the US, so that Bill could tell others about the possibilities of travelling to India (and to Icon in particular) for care: 'Now this person who had a culture shock coming to this hospital in this city in this part of the world, *he* is the one who gives confidence to the patients there [in the US].' The hospital room, then, operates in part as a laboratory for affective stumbles and repairs that become marked as 'culture' and that can be leveraged to attract future patients.

During an exchange of goodbyes the afternoon before Bill's surgery, a room attendant brought in two Pepsis for Bill and Judy. Bill raised himself on the bed and said:

> I don't know how much research you've done on hospitals, but over in the US, people that pay cash for their visits have to pay more than people with insurance, because we have to pay for the ones that don't pay. For the freeloaders in the US. The people that pay their bills, we have to pay for it. And I don't think that's right at all.

With this charge, Bill pushed aside the farce of rubles and rupees to open the space of the hospital room to critique. At stake was the configuration of American healthcare that impelled his decision to travel, and his position as an uninsured American who pays for the 'freeloaders' with either private insurance or government-funded Medicare. In a 'cashless' space of care, he and Judy had understanding listeners in Icon caregivers like Gautham as they reflected on their journey by tying cost and treatment comparisons to differences in sights, smells, and ways of social interaction. Gautham's hope for Bill and Judy was that upon their return, they would share the sentiments generated through their journey as a sales pitch for India and for Icon. Affect in this circumstance is a relational resource that can travel beyond its space of genesis, through a commitment ignited between patients, caregivers, and everyday objects like cash or food. Bill and Judy's case illustrates one pathway to this commitment, via encounters whose elements of awkwardness and humour trigger political critique. Icon's profit depends on this critique, but the trepidation and confusion that form it could potentially cast the Jacksons as figures of incredulity and naiveté, and the springboard for fear-fuelled accounts of medical travel like those of Glenn Beck or Robin Cook. Judy was aware of these stakes. 'People think we're crazy or just plain stupid,' she said of how the neighbours back home judged their decision to travel to India. But she deemed them less pressing than her immediate concern, pointing to Bill in the bed with a Pepsi in her hand, and showing how prior and future entailments lingered over the measure of their journey's success.

Touching lives

On another visit to Icon, Pooja, an international patient care 'hospitality officer,' made introductions to Mark, a barrister from London in his late 50s who had been in the hospital for nearly six weeks for spine surgery. While Mark ambled over to say hello, a nurse came into the room to take his blood pressure. Cuff on his arm, he grinned: 'You see, this is just how they all are – the help is unbelievable.' The nurse hushed him with a wagging finger so she could get a reading.

Over the course of several meetings together, Mark narrated his back injury in detail, beginning with the car crash in France he believed was its cause, and emphasised his 20 years of chronic pain. The accident gradually reconfigured his life: 'Everything becomes the pain.' His pain became so severe that he was unable to socialise, or to even sit down for dinner. Nor could he play with his children, whose photos were taped around his hospital bed. His wife eventually left him: 'You deteriorate as you go along, and people start saying you're boring,' he said. This was several years ago. His pain was deemed 'in his head' by his doctors in London, and despite his protests, he couldn't get on an expedited list for an MRI. He learned about Icon from a friend, and had an MRI within a day of arriving to India:

> The second night I was here, it was 1:30am and I was awake and they asked if I wanted my MRI done, and I said yippee, and they stuck me in the bloody wheelchair and took me downstairs. You wait half an hour, they do so many, over and over. In the UK I would've waited 8 or 9 months, maybe more, for something I've been waiting for, for years and years.

The doctors at Icon eventually found and removed spurs in his spine that Mark insists his doctors in the UK had missed for 20 years.

'This place is very well equipped,' Mark said assuredly. 'Did anyone tell you about the TV?' Mark asked Pooja to turn on the television, and the black screen fizzled and expanded to what looked like an infomercial about Icon. Mark said it was on continuous repeat, and he wound up watching it often at night when he couldn't sleep. Backgrounded by jovial Muzak, testimonial after testimonial from patients attested to the 'magic' of Icon's services on the screen. A distinguished older man came into the frame, explaining the history of Icon with hands confidently folded. 'That's the CEO,' Pooja whispered. The words 'loving care' frequently were uttered in the montage. 'They're right, they're absolutely right,' Mark said matter-of-factly. 'You will not believe the love you get in this place.' On cue, still-shots of the testimonials froze into a mosaic of smiling doctors, patients, and nurses, while an American-accented female voice soared in song in the background:

> *Reach out and touch*
> *It's simply magical, knowing you have the power to heal.*
> *Every day, every night*
> *Saving lives by the minute ... touching lives!*

Mark kept his gaze fixed on the TV, and pointed to his arm: 'Look at my skin. I'm getting – look! – I'm getting goose bumps. Because it's true.' Icon's invocations of love, magic, and salvation were visceral to him. These were not empty promises, he said. He *felt* them in his daily interactions. 'They all speak to you with such courtesy,' Mark noted. 'We'd like this sort of stuff to be in the West a bit, wouldn't we? We'd like people to behave like that a bit on our shores, instead of behaving as we see them on the telly, and the rap videos.'

Channel Icon became an interactive backdrop for the remainder of the time spent together, and reinforced the centrality of the television to the room's affective atmosphere. Mark would offer insights into his condition ('I've been in pain for over 20 years, I've been taking 14 painkillers a day'), and then a crisp feminine voice on the TV would croon an administrative tidbit ('Patients on Icon's package option are requested to deposit the specified amount in full upon admission'). It seemed impossible to sidestep the intense sense of care at Icon, found in the hospital's slogan of 'Touching Lives' printed on bed sheets and dishes, or materialized in the constant warm, focused attention. Nurses, staff, and doctors all stopped by to greet Mark, and he took several photos with them. Later in the day, in reflecting on Mark's case, a public relations staff member told me, 'Icon's people and services...it's quality care with a human touch...it's just machines and people, but it's definitely the kind of tender loving care which is extended to patients which makes the world of difference.' The intimacy of Icon's care and its incorporation as touch reinforced India's power to set right the affective entailments of foreign injuries.

To Mark, this form of healing intersected directly with his perspective on global flows of capital and power. During early moments of talking about medical tourism, he casually mentioned that he was 'anti-globalization' and that 'globalization is another stick that beats the poor'. When prompted to elaborate, he settled into his custom-fit back support chair ('they brought it especially for me'), and pointed to a stack of books on the desk:

> See, I've got these books on globalization, one that I'm giving to Gautham. I was actually going to do a thesis on it, and it was going to be called 'Globalization or the New Colonization?' or something like that. You're colonizing people via trade agreements, whereby you go into their countries, you rape them of their labour, pay them a pittance. I mean, yeah, I'm in India, I'm shocked at the price I'm paying. See, colonization was all about economy, it was about some people from one country going to another country, because they wanted to make loads of money. They wanted their gold, they wanted their spices, they wanted whatever they could get out of them. And then you have the example of India, where a company, I call it the biggest company take-over in the world, The East India Company took over the whole bloody country.

Mark continued on, mentioning the vicissitudes of Coke, McDonalds, and Starbucks invading 'the hearts and minds of the populace'. When asked what he thought about Americans who came to India for medical care, he scoffed:

> The richest country in the world has a system that forces dying people to go work to get treatment for terminal illnesses, when they're spending billions of dollars obliterating other societies, whether by globalization, or by funding roads in Afghanistan, or funding warlords who are running the cocaine industry.

Mark thought that Icon had found a way to use medical tourism to its advantage, enabling the treatment it gave to foreigners to be an avenue for caring for sick Indians. 'I think that what's happening is that we're paying for their people,' he said. 'Because the whole ethos of Icon is to give service with a smile, and to make you better.' There was a circuit of service at play in his analysis of the broader healthcare framework in India. Icon gave foreigners love, foreigners gave Icon money, and the money would translate into medical care for sick Indians. The atmosphere of care in the room trumped Mark's critiques of the rapacious nature of globalization. By connecting this space imaginatively to both past and contemporary spaces of coloniality, he envisioned its trickle-down possibilities to underwrite the broader healthcare system in India.

On Mark's last day at Icon, his room buzzed with doctors and nurses taking photos with him and saying their good-byes. The room was filled was a cool, metallic smell from the topical analgesic he sprayed on himself. After the room emptied out, he shared his feelings about leaving India. He said that he was always worried about having spine surgery, wherever it might take place. But after arriving in India and deeming Icon's surgeons 'very competent' and its facility top-notch, he surrendered: 'I just said, you do what you want, I'm the layperson.' Interrupting him, the electricity in the room cut out and the hum of the generator switched on. Channel Icon (now running on backup power) filled the pause in conversation. Soon after, Gautham called the room to thank Mark for the book about globalization. 'I hope you enjoy it', Mark replied. 'That book is very interesting for what you're doing.' He hung up, and said:

> You can write a song about it, a poem about it. All I can say is that the fact is, I came here, they found something wrong, and within a week I had surgery, and because I had so much pain...the pain was distorting my body's view of pain...as far as they're concerned it was small, but my body feels different.

Mark's pain was the touchstone for his recent life, and his visit to Icon opened up new possibilities for that life to become pain-free. He embodied his care at Icon, from the goose bumps of the infomercial to a cooling Ayurvedic sandalwood paste he was bringing back with him to London. Critical as he was of globalization, even locating medical tourism in its scope, Mark insisted that medical travel was a public good for India because it conveyed the 'loving care' of corporate medicine. Icon transformed his body, after freeing him from what he called a prison-like situation of doctors in the UK's National Health Service who concluded that he was imagining his pain, and who prevented him from getting the one diagnostic tool – the MRI – that might yield a remedy. In his analysis, colonization and globalization may be all about economy, but medical tourism (and Icon specifically) was about care, love, and healing, and offered an intimate antidote to suffering.

The promise

Medical tourism offers the promise of escape and repair to patients in dire healthcare straits. In India, the journey often crystallizes within the circumscribed spaces of the corporate hospital – spaces exemplary of the very form of market healthcare deemed to be hopeless in places like the US. Foreign patients in India reflected diverse sentiments: a sense of betrayal by their home countries, often in the register of an escape from restriction; a sense of being off-centre amidst stark differences in India; and a sense of comfort and deep gratitude to their Indian caregivers. Satisfaction over differences in cost and a sense of India tethered to loving care became medical tourism's salient features, as the affective journey of medical travel reanimated the parable of a foreigner who travels to a strange land filled with uncertainties (Pfeiffer 2002). Through the arc of an affective journey, a politics of repair coheres in these narratives by joining together patient subjectivity, risk, healthcare costs, and cultural difference. Affect serves as one channel for what Sherine Hamdy terms the 'political etiologies' of disease: how patients 'explain their disease etiology and illness experience as outcomes of social and political failures' (Hamdy 2008, 554). Judgements that patients make in India constantly tack back and forth to prior injuries, missed opportunities, and present possibilities, and unfold in the hospital room as a chronicle of ordinary sentiments.

What sort of ethical horizons extend from such politics? As Nancy Scheper-Hughes (2005, 164) asks about the organ trade, 'Are we witnessing the development of biosociality or the growth of a widespread bio-sociopathy?' For media outlets and marketers, globalization becomes a convenient, flimsy rationale for India's rise as a destination of medical care (Applbaum 2000; Mazzarella 2003). Many patients – even Mark with his invocations of colonialism and plunder – consistently landed on a refrain of rescue and relief, and not one of sociopolitical pathology. With few options available, medical tourism offered them a last-chance possibility of getting better. What was pathological, according to them and to their Indian caregivers, was their home healthcare systems whose shortcomings prompted the journey to India. Some patients expressed regret that their isolation in hospital rooms meant that there was little opportunity for them to critically assess everyday life and illness outside the hospital's walls. Very few planned on vacationing after treatment; most were like the Jacksons, who would be in Icon's care from the moment of arrival to departure.

In this sense, the affective spaces of the corporate hospital render other spaces invisible, like those in which Indians themselves turn to private facilities for care in lieu of the often gruff and harried treatment they receive at public clinics and hospitals strained by underfunding and administrative neglect (Das and Das 2006, 188). As Indian health activists have rightly asked: if public resources are funnelled to support corporate hospitals because of medical tourism's profit potential, what will become of public-sector facilities and the kinds of trade-offs their neglect instantiates? These issues merit further debate as medical travel increases, and this article has suggested that an ethnographic engagement with affect can articulate medical travel's problems and possibilities. The affective journey of medical travel encompasses 'countless intricately detailed little worlds built around major social injuries' (Stewart 2007, 43). It is in the spark of encounter where these injuries are found, and perhaps also where they can be eased.

Acknowledgements

This work was made possible by the patients, doctors, and hospital staff in India who shared their time and thoughts. The author is grateful to the Population Studies Training Center at Brown University for supporting the fieldwork portion of this project. The author thanks Catherine Lutz, Daniel J. Smith, Lina Fruzzetti, Stephen Houston, João Biehl, Charles Briggs, Lawrence Cohen, Joseph Dumit, Margaret Lock, Ashis Nandy, Sunil Nandraj and Gabriel Rosenberg for their tremendous guidance. The author also thanks Cristiana Bastos, Harish Naraindas, and two anonymous *A&M* reviewers for their engaged critique and support, although the presentation of ideas here is his own.

Ethics: This project received approval from the Brown University Research Protections Office.

Funding: Population Studies Training Center, Brown University.

Conflict of interest: none.

Notes

1. 'Medical tourism' and 'medical travel' are used interchangeably in this paper to balance the discursive ubiquity of the term 'medical tourism' in Indian media with the term 'medical travel' used in social science scholarship. In interviews, most patients expressed that the vacation element of medical travel was irrelevant if not ridiculous. See Inhorn and Patrizio (2009) and Sobo (2009) on terminology.
2. All names used here, both personal and institutional, are pseudonyms unless noted otherwise.
3. See Ahmed (2004) and Ducey (2007) on emotion, value, and capital.
4. Also see Berlant (2000), Clough and Halley (2007), Mazzarella (2009), and Thrift (2007) for in-depth explorations of 'the affective turn.'

5. See Lefebvre (2008) on the rise of corporate hospitals in urban India.
6. The notion of 'cost advantage' attached to Indian medicine is not new, as historian of science Shamshad Khan points out (2006).
7. The actual numbers reported of travelling patients vary; a common figure is 150,000 international patients coming to India each year, of which Europeans and Americans constitute a small (but growing) percentage, but can vary up to one million, exemplifying what Jean and John Comaroff call 'quantifacts', figures whose 'assertions of the real . . . fill the space between the unknowable and the axiomatic, imagination and anxiety' (Comaroff and Comaroff 2006, 209).
8. The paper's focus is on biomedicine (sometimes called 'allopathic medicine' in India), although there is a significant amount of medical tourism for local healing modalities such as Ayurveda.
9. The author visited several branches of this hospital chain across India, but for the purposes of simplicity each hospital is referred to as its parent company name.
10. This evokes Gay Becker's (2007, 302) notion of 'containment' whereby US health insurance policies marginalize people without insurance. For explorations of these stakes outside the US, particularly following neoliberal restructuring of national health services, see Biehl (2005), Das (2003), and Rylko-Bauer and Farmer (2002).
11. Judy's actions illustrate Gay Becker's emphasis that uninsured Americans are not passive agents in the process of containment, and defy the hotel-like leisure indicated by the term 'concierge'.
12. Icon has since solidified partnerships with several insurance companies, including Blue Cross/Blue Shield and CIGNA.

References

Adams, V., M. Murphy, and A. Clarke. 2009. Anticipation: Technoscience, life, affect, temporality. *Subjectivity* 28, no. 1: 246–65.

Ahmed, S. 2004. Affective economies. *Social Text* 22, no. 2: 117–39.

Ananthakrishnan, G. 2006. Boom time for medicare. *The Hindu*, April 30, Magazine.

Applbaum, K. 2000. Crossing borders: Globalization as myth and charter in American transnational consumer marketing. *American Ethnologist* 27, no. 2: 257–82.

Augé, M. 1985. Interpreting illness. *History and Anthropology* 2, no. 1: 1–13.

Baru, R. 2005. Private health sector in India: Raising inequities. In *Review of Healthcare in India*, ed. L. Gangolli, Ravi Duggal, and Abhay Shukla. Mumbai: Center for Enquiry into Health & Allied Themes (CEHAT).

Beck, G. 2009. The Glenn Beck program, 9 December 2009.

Becker, G. 2007. The uninsured and the politics of containment in U.S. health care. *Medical Anthropology* 26, no. 4: 299–321.

Berlant, L. 2000. *Intimacy*. Chicago: University of Chicago Press.

Bhardwaj, A. 2008. Biosociality and biocrossings: Encounters with assisted conception and embryonic stem cells in India. In *Biosocialities, Genetics, and the Social Sciences: Making Biologies and Identities*, ed. Sahra Gibbon and Carlos Novas, New York: Routledge.

Biehl, J. 2005. *Vita: Life in a zone of social abandonment*. Berkeley: University of California Press.

Biehl, J., D. Coutinho, and A.L. Outeiro. 2001. Technology and affect: HIV/AIDS testing in Brazil. *Culture, Medicine and Psychiatry* 25, no. 1: 87–129.

Clough, P., and J. Halley, eds. 2007. *The affective turn: Theorizing the social*. Durham: Duke University Press.

Cohen, L. 1995. The epistemological carnival: Meditations on disciplinary intentionality and Ayurveda. In *Knowledge and the scholarly medical traditions*, ed. D. Bates, Cambridge: Cambridge University Press.

Comaroff, J., and J. Comaroff. 2006. Figuring crime: Quantifacts and the production of the un/real. *Public Culture* 18, no. 1: 209–45.

Confederation of Indian Industry (CII). 2002. *Healthcare in India: The road ahead.* New Delhi: Confederation of Indian Industry.

Cook, R. 2008. *Foreign body.* New York: Putnam.

Das, V., and R.K. Das. 2006. Pharmaceuticals in urban ecologies: The register of the local. In *Global Pharmaceuticals: Ethics, Markets, Practices,* ed. Adriana Petryna, Andrew Lakoff and Arthur Kleinman, Durham: Duke University Press.

Das, V. 2003. Technologies of self: Poverty and health in an urban setting. *SARAI Reader.* 95–102. New Delhi: SARAI.

Ducey, A. 2007. More than a job: Meaning, affect, and training health care workers. In *The affective turn: Theorizing the social,* ed. Patricia T. Clough and Jean Halley. Durham: Duke University Press.

Duggal, R. 1996. *The private health sector in India: Nature, trends, and a critique.* Mumbai: Centre for Enquiry into Health and Allied Themes (CEHAT).

Government of India. National Health Policy. 2002. http://mohfw.nic.in/np2002.htm.

Gray, H.H., and S.C. Poland. 2008. Medical tourism: Crossing borders to access health care. *National Reference Center for Bioethics Literature* SCOPE, note 47.

Hamdy, S.F. 2008. When the state and your kidneys fail: Political etiologies in an Egyptian dialysis ward. *American Ethnologist* 35, no. 4: 553–69.

Haniffa, A. 2009. Indian-American organisations slam Glenn Beck. Rediff News. http://news.rediff.com/report/2009/dec/17/indian-american-organisations-slam-glenn-beck-for-comments.htm

Henry J. Kaiser Family Foundation. 2008. Health insurance coverage in America, 2008. Henry J. Kaiser Family Foundation. http://facts.kff.org/chartbook.aspx?cb = 57

Hochschild, A. 2003. *The managed heart: Commercialization of human feeling.* Berkeley: University of California Press.

Iedema, R., C. Jorm, and M. Lum. 2009. Affect is central to patient safety: The horror stories of young anaesthetists. *Social Science & Medicine* 69: 1750–56.

Inhorn, M., and P. Patrizio. 2009. Rethinking reproductive 'tourism' as reproductive 'exile'. *Fertility and Sterility* 92, no. 3: 904–6.

Kangas, B. 2002. Therapeutic itineraries in a global world: Yeminis and their search for biomedical treatment abroad. *Medical Anthropology* 21: 35–78.

Kangas, B. 2007. Hope from abroad in the international medical travel of Yemeni patients. *Anthropology & Medicine* 14, no. 3: 293–305.

Khan, S. 2006. Systems of medicine and nationalist discourse in India: towards 'new horizons' in medical anthropology and history. *Social Science & Medicine* 62: 2786–97.

Latour, B. 2005. *Reassembling the social: An introduction to actor-network theory.* Oxford: Oxford University Press.

Lefebvre, B. 2008. The Indian corporate hospitals: Touching middle class lives. In *Patterns of middle class consumption in India and China,* ed. Christophe Jaffrelot and Peter van der Veer. London: Sage.

Lutz, C. 1986. Emotion, thought, and estrangement: Emotion as a cultural category. *Cultural Anthropology* 1, no. 3: 287–309.

Lutz, C., and G. White. 1986. The anthropology of emotions. *Annual Review of Anthropology* 15, no. 1: 405–36.

Mazzarella, W. 2003. *Shoveling smoke: Advertising and globalization in contemporary India.* Durham: Duke University Press.

Mazzarella, W. 2009. Affect: What is it good for? In *Enchantments of modernity: Empire, nation, globalization,* ed. Saurabh Dube, New Delhi: Routledge.

Navaro-Yashin, Y. 2009. Affective spaces, melancholic objects: Ruination and the production of anthropological knowledge. *Journal of the Royal Anthropological Institute (NS)* 15: 1–18.

Patel, G. 2007. Imagining risk, care, and security: Insurance and fantasy. *Anthropological Theory* 7, no. 1: 99–117.

Pfeiffer, J. 2002. African independent churches in Mozambique: Healing the afflictions of inequality. *Medical Anthropology Quarterly* 16, no. 2: 176–99.

Roberts, E.F.S. Forthcoming. Disease and destination: Medical travel before the contagious age. *Body & Society*.

Rylko-Bauer, B., and P. Farmer. 2002. Managed care or managed inequality? A call for critiques of market-based medicine. *Medical Anthropology Quarterly* 16, no. 4: 476–502.

Scheper-Hughes, N. 2005. The last commodity: Post-human ethics and the global traffic in 'fresh' organs. In *Global assemblages: Technology, politics, and ethics as anthropological problems*, ed. Aihwa Ong and Steven Collier, Oxford: Blackwell.

Sengupta, A. 2008. Medical tourism in India: Winners and losers. *Indian Journal of Medical Ethics* 5, no. 1.

Sengupta, A., and Samiran Nundy. 2005. The private health sector in India is burgeoning, but at the cost of public health care. *British Medical Journal* 331: 1157–8.

Sobo, E.J. 2009. Medical travel: What it means, why it matters. *Medical Anthropology* 28, no. 4: 326–35.

Song, P. 2010. Biotech pilgrims and the transnational quest for stem cell cures. *Medical Anthropology* 29, no. 4: 384–402.

Stewart, K. 2007. *Ordinary affects*. Durham: Duke University Press.

Stoler, A.L. 2002. *Carnal knowledge and imperial power: Race and the intimate in colonial rule*. Berkeley: University of California Press.

Sunder Rajan, K. 2006. *Biocapital: The constitution of postgenomic life*. Durham: Duke University Press.

Thrift, N. 2007. *Non-representational theory: Space, politics, affect*. New York: Routledge.

Whittaker, A. 2008. Pleasure and pain: Medical travel in Asia. *Global Public Health* 3, no. 3: 271–90.

Whittaker, A. 2009. Global technologies and transnational reproduction in Thailand. *Asian Studies Review* 33, no. 3: 319–32.

Selling medical travel to US patient-consumers: the cultural appeal of website marketing messages

Elisa J. Sobo, Elizabeth Herlihy and Mary Bicker

San Diego State University, San Diego, California, USA

More US-based patients than ever are travelling abroad for medical or dental services. Beyond financial incentives, what cultural factors have supported this trend? Because of their interest in selling medical travel, medical travel agencies (MTAs) have vested interests in this question. To find out how they are answering it, an ethnographic content analysis of MTA websites was undertaken. Beyond themes promoting a 'worry-free experience' of 'legitimate services', themes linking healthcare consumerism to culturally specific identity ideals and self-creation/representation processes predominated. Themes relating to the demonstration of social position, savvy expression of good consumer judgment, and achievement of libertarian ideals figured highly. However, various inconsistencies (including an appeal to tourism in some but not other situations) suggested that medical travel involves, for the US-based consumer, a complex act of juggling context-specific self-identity desires and expectations in relation to healthcare. The potential impact of prevailing discourses on 'self-construction-in-practice' was explored. Findings enhance understanding of the care seeking process as experienced within the context of globalized, mass-mediated healthcare consumerism. They also point to the need for finer-grained distinctions than the global gloss 'medical travel' offers.

Introduction

Travel for the primary purpose of obtaining medical or dental services is on the rise. Some reasons for this are financial and technological – but, as in other realms of medicine, cultural features also must play a role in fostering demand. Medical travel agencies or MTAs (i.e., their owners and those who manage and staff them) have vested interests in sharply perceiving and leveraging these features to corner the market. An examination of strategies undertaken by MTAs to do so can broaden knowledge regarding the cultural context in which US consumers consider and undertake medical travel. To this end, an 'ethnographic content analysis' (Altheide, 1987) of MTA websites targeting the USA was undertaken.

The study's findings enhance understanding of care-seeking processes as experienced within the context of globalization and in light of the rise of consumerism as a major tenet in US culture. They illuminate themes prevalent in the decision to outsource one's healthcare, and elucidate the self-construction practices and aims implicated. By focusing on medical travel facilitators rather than producers or consumers, this study highlights a generally overlooked yet potentially crucial part of the medical travel marketplace. And by incorporating the internet, the research has great relevance for scholars seeking to adequately understand contemporary social life and self-construction (cf. Garcia et al. 2009; e.g. Altheide 2000; Holstein and Gubrium 2000).

Background

The global business of medicine

In part due to 'the liberalization of trade in services, the growing cooperation between private and public sectors, the easy global spread of information about products and services, and, most importantly, the successful splicing of the tourism and health sectors' (Bookman and Bookman 2007, 95), more patients outbound from various North American and European nations have joined the medical travel consumer population. In the USA, thanks to (among other things) high numbers of un- and under-insured individuals; an increasing demand for so-called lifestyle care, such as knee replacements and aesthetic or cosmetic surgery; technological developments supporting quicker, less invasive surgeries; increased awareness of options due to word-of-mouth (including internet discussions); and increased general media coverage of the phenomenon, the number of medical travellers is growing year by year (Keckley and Underwood 2008, 3).

Asian nations are among those that have actively pursued medical travellers as well as programmatically encouraging necessary infrastructural development (Whittaker 2008, 275).[1] Hotelmarketing.com estimates that 'the industry in Malaysia, Thailand, Singapore and India, currently worth around half a billion dollars a year in Asia, is projected to generate more than US$4.4 billion by 2012. India's medical tourism business is growing at 30 per cent per year' (Anonymous 2006). Similarly rosy prognostications abound.

While some outbound travellers seek treatments unavailable in the USA, the majority of medical travel has been explained by financial logic: a hip replacement costs about $37,000 in the USA and $13,000 in India. An $80,000 US heart bypass is $16,000 in Thailand (Higgins 2007). Using weighted average procedure prices, one report put the average savings from the US perspective at about 85% (Keckley and Underwood 2008, 13). Although in many reports financial logic speaks for itself, it only can do so in light of pervasive US beliefs that healthcare is a market good and that patients are (capable) consumers.

Beyond its financial logic, care procured at certified non-US facilities is generally of equal or better quality than the US standard (Milstein and Smith 2006). This appeals in the cultural context of consumer advocacy and provider accountability. One source of information on quality is the Joint Commission International (JCI), organized by the US-based Joint Commission, which accredits US healthcare organizations. Other organizations, such as the International Society for Quality in Health care (ISQUA), also have participated in accreditation efforts. Quality is assured through a number of processes, including use of evidence-based clinical guidelines, provision of care plans to patients for facilitation self-care, electronic medical record and clinical information systems, coordination of care with a patient's home-town providers, adverse event action plans, outcomes measurement and reporting, etc (Keckley and Underwood 2008, 8–9).

Consequently, some US insurance companies (such as BlueCross BlueShield of South Carolina) and government payers (such as the state of West Virginia) have considered sending patients overseas for certain types of care, or offering them cash rebates for doing so (Bramstedt and Xu 2007; Carrol 2007). In California, several insurance companies now offer bi-national (US-Mexico) coverage.

Anthropological views

Beyond attending to its various political-economic dimensions for critical purposes (e.g., Scheper-Hughes 2002), existing anthropological literature on medical travel has generally focused on the medical travel consumer. Most scholars have been interested in how consumers use (or strive to use) medical travel to meet particular cultural expectations.

For example, Beth Kangas, a pioneer in the area, has studied travel from Yemen undertaken (when possible) for cancer and other care unavailable there. Kangas has shown that Yemenite families send relatives abroad for care as a public demonstration of affection or 'to prove that they did everything they could for their loved ones' (Kangas 2002, p. 66) as well as to avoid criticism for not doing so, and to deflect attributions of culpability for a relative's demise onto the medical system (see also Kangas 2007). In addition to its physical benefits, then, medical travel is crucial in how people create and maintain their identities as 'good' relatives (e.g., parents, spouses, children).

While Kangas has focused on people with problems such as cancer, other work to date has been concerned with travel for reproductive procedures. (e.g., Inhorn and Patrizio 2009; Speier 2008; and see Inhorn and see Speier, this issue). Identity and social role fulfilment issues remain a prominent theoretical focus. Particular questions relate to the relationship between gendered reproductive ideals and cultural and socio-political citizenship, status, and authority. The antagonism between the kind of corporeal partibility supported by market logic and the ideal of bodily integrity, the rise of consumer-oriented medicine in general, and the critique of US biomedicine implicit in much outbound medical travel also has been of concern.

Cosmetic or aesthetically-motivated medical travel also has garnered a share of research attention; here, self-production displaces reproduction but otherwise similar concerns surface. Sara Ackerman, for example, conducted ethnographic interviews of cosmetic surgery seekers in Costa Rica (Ackerman n.d.). While her main focus was the social divisions manifest in and reinforced by the plastic surgery trade, most consumers to whom she spoke were quite self-concerned. Further, most cast the decision for alteration as part of a holistically restorative process. Cosmetic surgery was seen as a form of mind-body realignment or repair, in which an inner 'self' that had become disjointed from a person's (often younger, or ideal) body was reunited with the body that it deserved or to which it was already once connected. Cosmetic surgery, from this perspective, is the opposite of frivolous. It provides for 'full social participation, or citizenship' (Ackerman n.d.).

Questions raised

While there is much to be learned directly from consumers, it also makes sense to query the various organizational or institutional contexts for their actions. Doing so can reveal both the structural and discursive constraints delimiting their actions, and the desires and understandings they bring to the endeavour, at least inasmuch as the contexts reflect them. In this regard, scrutiny of medical travel facilitation organizations is ideal.

Whether for profit or service motives, medical travel agencies or MTAs (i.e., their owners and those who manage and staff them) have vested interests in attaining a keen understanding of consumer concerns and desires: they want to leverage this understanding to meet consumer needs and/or sell their goods. Assuming they have got an at least fairly accurate reading of their market (it is in their best interests to do so), an examination of the themes articulated on their sites, and the ways these themes are deployed in the quest to produce actual customers, can broaden knowledge regarding the cultural context in which US consumers consider and undertake medical travel. So too can information regarding whether and how internal differentiation of the US medical travel market (for instance for oncology vs. procreative vs. aesthetic services, etc) is reflected in MTA website discourse.

There is another reason for querying MTA websites. Existing research on medical travel highlights issues related to self-construction, self-perception, and self-presentation that consumers find salient. Further scrutiny may help advance understanding in this area.[2]

For example, the 'self' referenced by Ackerman's participants seems to be what Victor de Munck elsewhere has shown as a culturally constructed 'self symbol' – one that not only reflects cultural ideals but also provides an 'illusion of a unified, coherent self' (de Munck 1992, 167). This illusion veils a multiplicity of identities and associated 'subselves,' each including particular 'behavioural, cognitive, and affective complexes' (de Munck 1992, 171). Participants in Ackerman's work would have subjectively experienced regeneration through reintegration both because of their culturally constructed expectations for 'self' (including self-coherence) and in spite of the incoherence that the 'self' serves to mask.

The 'self' may a symbol be but, as Holstein and Gubrium (2000, 12) note, it is 'widely produced' in keeping with the contemporary cultural (including institutional) demand for it: it is 'something persons must continually manifest as a basis for making sense of their conduct and relationships'. For Holstein and Gubrium, self-construction is an ongoing, practical, every-day, contingent, context-based 'interpretive practice' (Holstein and Gubrium 2000, 94) and a lot of work goes into this. People are not each on their own, however. People participate in myriad institutions or 'going concerns' (Holstein and Gubrium 2000, 13, citing Hughes 1984). Furthermore, 'Selves are themselves institutional projects in the sense that institutional discourses provide the conditions of possibility and institutionalized discursive practice supplies the model of production for putting into effect our identities as part of accomplishing matters of ongoing local interest' (Holstein and Gubrium 2000, 95).

In light of this, and in light of the increasing numbers of medical travellers, in addition to seeking to catalogue MTAs' understanding of consumer concerns and desires, research might also ask what 'model of production' or self template medical travel agency (MTA) websites are providing. As these questions involve cultural meanings, an ethnographically informed approach will work best.

Methods

To address the issues at hand, an 'ethnographic[3] content analysis' (Altheide 1987) was undertaken of MTA websites: cultural artefacts created by the medical travel industry. This approach entails a reflexive, iterative engagement with documents; the 'constant comparison' technique (Glaser and Strauss 1967) is dominant. The investigator plays a central role, moving back and forth reflexively between, as per Altheide's list, 'concept development, sampling, data collection, data coding, data analysis, and interpretation' (Altheide 1987, 68). Recall that consumers' imagined presence and real feedback provided by them to MTAs play a huge role in shaping the artefacts under analysis – just as the 'going concern' of the MTA provides an institutional context for shaping consumer selves. Ethnographic content analysis findings therefore can reveal much more than just what the media 'contain'.

Sampling strategy

'MTA website' was defined as a website intended to sell comprehensive medical travel services, which are not only clinical services but also transportation, accommodation, and pre- and post-procedural assistance. To limit focus, further eligibility was limited to MTAs with offices in the USA and websites in English.

To ensure a broad sampling universe, searchenginewatch.com was consulted for the latest search engine rankings released by comScore (Gunasekera, Ernst, and Ezra 2008). The research used the top three which, together, accounted for 91% of all internet searches (Burns 2008). The search term 'medical tourism' was selected as it produced the highest number of eligible MTA 'hits' in feasibility tests (regarding scholarly objections to this label, see Sobo 2009; see also Inhorn and Patrizio 2009; Kangas, 2010).

To amass a sample that would provide ample data for valid and reliable findings, for each search engine, each of the first 150 hits that met the eligibility criteria described was collected, leading to 49 eligible websites. Twenty-seven were unique. Because 'the World Wide Web is a fast-moving medium' (van Esch, Cornel, and Snoek, 2006, 1235), each website's pages were printed for static storage and data stability, with colour and animation information noted as relevant.

Building the codebook and coding website content

The websites were randomized and divided for inductive code development. Coding focused not only on prevalent ideas or 'themes' (content) but also, following Norris et al. (2006), the structural characteristics (form; e.g. colour palate, organizational features) of the various websites. The research's main goal was to build a conceptual map or model of MTA ideas about potential customers directly from, or grounded in and traceable to, the texts under study (Glaser and Strauss 1967; Strauss and Corbin 1998). As ethnographic content analysis is a reflexive process (Altheide 1987), the final model was also influenced by what the researchers saw during preliminary sampling trials as well as by literature regarding the US healthcare consumer movement and, in regard to structural codes, by their knowledge of basic website architecture.

The search for themes began with 'open coding' (Glaser and Strauss 1967), in which all three authors (the research team members) closely reviewed the websites through iterative, recursive reading with the aim of identifying and labelling variables. Team members independently reviewed their allocated websites to the point of saturation (i.e., when the texts became redundant). Each took careful notes on all discrete ideas about medical travel mentioned, bearing in mind the situation-specific contexts in which they were brought up. Each attended to repetitions, metaphors and analogies, key words, transitions and syntactic connectors, indige-nous categories or typologies (e.g., ideas expressed colloquially), depiction of causal chains, evaluation claims, shifts from past to present tense, and digressions (Hill 2005; Quinn 2005; Ryan and Bernard 2003). Each compared like examples across websites and looked for disconfirming cases.

Each team member produced a preliminary set of data-grounded open codes. To best reflect the MTA point of view, code names were drawn directly from, or paraphrases of, language used in the websites.

The team met to compare code sets and then hone and merge them. The team then generated a codebook with, as is standard, one row for each code and four columns: one each for the code, its definition, an example, and any special rules.

MB and EH then reviewed website print-outs to extract data regarding structural features. They did this together as a quality assurance measure.

MB and EH began thematic coding also as a pair. Pair coding promotes reliability because it demands explicit vocalization of assumptions and regular cross-checks of the same as well as calling on paired investigators to regularly challenge each other's distinctions (Salinger, Plonka, and Prechelt 2008, 18). When agreement was secure, MB and EH split and individually coded the remaining websites. They met regularly with each other and ES to compare notes and ideas; troubleshoot any difficult passages, and reconfirm or realign code agreements. The codebook was refined by consensus, as needed. By the time the 15th website was coded, redundancy had clearly been realized and the codebook had long been stable. The formal analysis phase then began.

Thematic analysis

With the data at hand, each team member individually sorted the codes into groups representing the organizing principles implicated in MTA rhetoric. The team then came together to compare, discuss, reorder as deemed appropriate, and name the higher-order categories and relationships that emerged when the individual sorts were combined. Reference was made, as needed, to open-coding notes, and to the websites themselves (when questions related to context of use). Disconfirming cases and rival hypotheses regarding code categorization were sought out and explored.

A preliminary figure depicting the categories in relation to one another was mapped and then refined. MB and EH prepared summaries of every category and its subsumed themes, including for reference pertinent website passages.

As a final double-check, both MB and EH coded three more websites each, bringing the total number of coded websites to 21. No new codes or insights were noted, and no ideas generated on the basis of the initial 15 websites were disconfirmed.

In addition, to help assure validity, the team also sought periodic feedback from an MTA owner with whom the first author had previously worked. A second MTA worker recruited by the first corroborated the final summary of findings.

Findings

Key structural features of the 27 websites are shown in Table 1. Business names were fairly similar in the sample, referring generically to healthcare, global travel, and sometimes affordability.

Themes (codes, code categories) prominent on the websites fit into several higher-order groups that, as shown in Figure 1, supported a 'worry free experience', the MTAs' key good. This experience would be, first and foremost – as per the 'MTA promise' – 'world class', 'high quality', and 'affordable'. Themes illustrating with more detail how these overarching goals were to be achieved comprise three lower-order, goal-supporting category groups: 'self-production via consumption', 'all-inclusive patient care', and 'legitimate services'. The legend provides details regarding the figure's arrangement.

Table 1. Sample characteristics ($N = 27$).

Structural feature	Websites where present
Site map	16 (59%)
Dominant colour: Blue	21 (78%)*
Agency logo	27 (100%)
'Our Process' page	17 (63%)
Procedure information list	27 (100%)
Procedure information list with external links	05 (19%)
Cost comparison table	12 (44%)
FAQs	22 (81%)
Registration page: for individuals	11 (41%)
Registration page: for providers	03 (11%)
Page/area for payers (insurers)	10 (37%)
Page/area for providers	11 (41%)
'Contact us' dialogue page	27 (100%)
Terms and conditions information	18 (67%)
Links to media: Agency coverage	10 (37%)
Links to media: Medical travel (e.g., popularity of)	19 (70%)**
MTA update blog	07 (26%)
Patient testimonials – Written	19 (70%)
Patient testimonials – Video	09 (33%)
Marketing questionnaire	08 (30%)
Rotating photographs	15 (56%)
Photo emphasis on tourism vs. medicine	6 (22%)***

*Of these ($n = 21$), nine paired blue with white; four paired it with green; three with yellow; one with grey; and one with tan.
**52% of this was video coverage.
***The majority of frozen, sampled versions of the 27 websites (20; 74%) contained pictures emphasizing the medical aspect of medical travel (one had no emphasis).

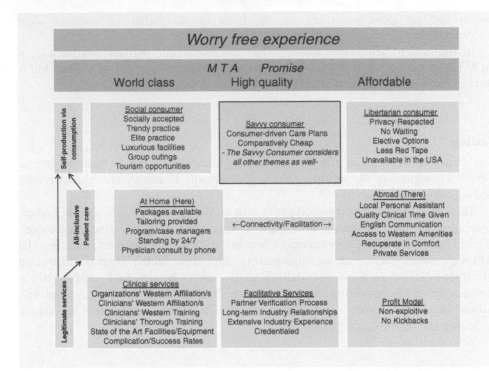

Figure 1. Visual depiction of themes and their overall organization in medical travel agency or MTA websites. Boxes contain coded themes, organized into categories (underlined). The spatial location of a given box or row of boxes reflects its position in website discourse on MTA services. Meta-themes are represented in the top two rows, with row two's general 'MTA promise' themes supporting the even more general promise of a 'worry free experience' (row one). The lower three rows (rows three-five) depict the categories whose themes reference details regarding how overarching promises will be achieved. Labels for these rows (groups of categories) are shown in column one, in boldface. 'Self-production via consumption' (row three) is central because it, and particularly its central category ('savvy consumer'), figured centrally in the analysis. The 'savvy consumer' is in fact produced with reference to or the support of all other themes and categories infusing the MTA websites. The arrows linking row (category group) labels, and the lower placement of rows four and five, map the 'savvy consumer' group's contingent or dependent relationship. The central, themeless category in row four ('connectivity/facilitation') links the two main aspects of 'all-inclusive care' together as well as being a key MTA industry product; and the bottom row depicts themes of legitimacy that are foundational to the whole enterprise. While themes denoted in the figure directly correspond to or paraphrase MTA messages, category (box) and category group (row) labels reflect underlying organizing principles, which generally remained implicit in the texts.

MTA promise

The most commonly mentioned themes on the MTA websites related to each MTA's driving intention to connect consumers with top-notch care at affordable prices. Websites made liberal use of catch-phrases indicating such (for example, 'Our primary aims to facilitate the highest standard of quality medical treatment and patient care at a cost which is affordable' [4.1; i.e. Website 4, page 1]). However, these phrases were under-defined. Themes in the supporting categories (see Figure 1's lower three rows) filled in the picture.

Legitimate services

Key to the MTA enterprise is the assertion that the services sold are legitimate. Through themes categorized under 'Clinical Services', MTAs represented offshore clinical care as the same if not better than the US standard. For example, one MTA offered 'hospitals which are JCI accredited and are affiliated with a branch of the prestigious Johns Hopkins University' [13.4]. This MTA further asserted that 'most of their physicians are educated in UK or US and are board certified' [13.8].

Several websites bolstered claims of affiliation and equivalence by directly referencing the international heritage of the current Western clinical workforce. For example, one asserted, 'In the USA, 1 out of 20 practicing doctors are Indians.... Indian doctors are found in almost all parts of the world.... Indians make up roughly 20 percent of the 'International Medical Graduates' – or foreign-trained doctors – operating in the US' [17.29].

In addition to highlighting Western affiliations and training, the thoroughness of clinician training and the state of the art facilities and technologies on offer were promoted. For instance, one hospital was advertised as 'equipped with cutting edge technology, digital flat panel cath labs, state of the art operating theatres' etc [5.23]. Also relevant were references to complication and success rates; for example, 'The death rate among patients during surgery is only 0.8 percent. This is less than half the equivalent rate in most major hospitals in the United States' [11.32].

In website discourse, MTA 'Facilitative Services' were represented as of the highest professional calibre. Many listed their credentials as members of the Better Business Bureau and Medical Tourism Association. Processes for verifying the legitimacy of providers/partners were explained (e.g. '[Our MTA] investigates every facet of a surgeon's credentials... Our process for choosing doctors takes an average of three months and generally only one surgeon out of thirty meet our strict requirements' [16.44]). Many claimed to have longstanding professional relationships within the industry, as well as extensive experience in the MTA field (e.g. 'We have over 20 years of experience running healthcare service companies and working with medical centers overseas 75 years' [5.5]), although quantitative data regarding how long a given agency had been in business was rarely provided.

The integrity of the MTA business itself was defended through reference to a 'Profit Model' that explicitly denied the exploitation of foreign workers or receipt of kickbacks. Prices were justified with reference to 'the lower cost of living [overseas], a strong dollar, and lower physician fees' [5.46], although some MTAs also noted that malpractice insurance costs, too, are lower outside of the USA (e.g. 3.1).

All-inclusive care

On top of legitimacy rhetoric, another layer of thematic content focused on positioning MTAs as able to offer 'all inclusive' service. This included travel packages or tailor-made itineraries.

The 'all inclusive' 'worry free experience' began 'At Home (Here)'. A program or case manager would 'work with you, making notes of your preferences, and with your cooperation and input, we will arrange a complete and comprehensive medical and travel package which includes all our customized services' [11.3]. In addition, 'Your US Case Manager will help you with your travel from home country to destination country in detail. They will provide you with valuable advice about rules and regulations, culture and what to expect' [9.5].

Both before and during medical travel, 'program managers are available 24/7 to serve you. They sleep with their cell phones so that they are in constant contact with you. You will never have to worry' [11.10]. Foreign physicians also are available by phone (sometimes with video): 'We can arrange for a "consultation conference call". The intention here is that you get to know the medical team and they understand more about your physical condition, required treatment and any personal history' [12.4]. There was no question that a personal relationship would be forged – one that extended beyond hospital and even national walls.

Round the clock care was not just clinical: Once overseas ('Abroad [There]'), 'You will be assigned a personal assistant who will meet you on arrival. This person will be your 'friend away from home' and is at your disposal during your stay. That person will accompany you to all medical appointments and will be with you pre- and post-operatively in the hospital' [16.45]. Some MTAs spoke, for instance, of 'transportation, translation, concierge service and more,' to be provided by this advocate [10.18].

Overseas clinicians are portrayed in the websites as able to spend significant quality clinical time with each patient, constantly checking in and making themselves available. In addition, clinicians simply are more numerous: 'The level of service in terms of nursing care is second to none with nurse-to-patient ratios approaching one-to-one' [5.3]. Further, communication will be in 'fluent English' [10.2] or, if not, via fluent interpreters. Access to Western amenities (e.g., television channels, coffee makers, in-room safes, familiar foods) is assured.

Also assured is privacy as well as comfort during recuperation. For example, in one facility, 'All rooms are newly renovated suites with an ocean view. This area is ideal for your recovery' [16.35]. In another, one may 'relax and recuperate in idyllic surroundings' [11.31]. This type of setting, sold as fostering healing, is opposed in website discourse to settings in which recovery is rushed, surroundings unpleasant, roommates unavoidable, iatrogenic infections expectable, and access to nurses and other clinicians delayed or difficult.

Self-production via consumption

Throughout the medical travel process, in addition to the body work surgery and other procedures involve, consumers can work on bolstering a specific type of self-image. For instance, consumers engage in practices that reinforce a 'social' self-image. Medical travel is sold as a socially acceptable option: 'hundreds of thousands of people annually are exploring the advantages of medical tourism' [16.10]. Many MTAs referred to validating media coverage as (e.g. 'But as FOX 26's Melissa Wilson reports' [1.11]). Medical travel was sold as part of a new, 'trendy' movement, with today's medical traveller on the leading edge of a popular 'rush' [11.23].

Of course, as MTAs note, 'the global elite have been travelling [for care] for years' [12.8]'. Today, MTAs can connect everyone with clinics 'where the rich and famous have been going' [12.58]. When people 'realize they can afford VIP treatment...they're packing their bags' to partake in '"lifestyles of the rich and famous" treatment' [16.10]. Thus, through medical travel, common consumers join the ranks of 'high profile corporate clients' [12.14], a 'well-known Dallas socialite' [16.10], and so on. They, too, are accommodated in luxury, for instance 'at a 4 or

5 star hotel' [4.7]. Customers have access to 'premier packages with extensive customized luxuries' [11.3]. Promoting customers' alignment with people of value, the MTAs 'take an active role in bringing you the healthcare you need and deserve' [7.2].

Luxuries to be deservingly indulged include not only the facilities but also local sights. One website promised 'an exotic tourist destination with plenty of beaches, mountains, rivers and greenery to enjoy' [13.23]. Another noted, 'Some medical tourists spend a few days sightseeing before their procedures while others enjoy the same while recuperating' [1.24]. Some mentioned the option of making medical travel a sociable group event: 'Are you considering travelling with more than two people to same destination for medical treatment? Our group discount package is designed to accommodate your needs' [10.51].

Another marketing angle is an appeal to healthcare consumerism in which self-empowered customers make savvy choices, actively self-managing their care. For instance, one Website 'empowers you to take charge of your health' [10.1]; another's 'intention is to provide you with all possible information on the hospitals and surgeons for you to make an informed decision' [7.43]. Not the doctor's order but the consumer's choice drives a medical travel booking.

Customers are encouraged to discuss options with their local providers; however, when given, this directive generally has a rote, legalistic feeling, as if a mandated disclaimer. Statements reinforcing consumer agency and emphasizing the MTA's role in assisting and enabling consumers to make their own choices dominate. Websites assert that consumers will 'gather as much information as possible' [11.31] in their quest for the best possible care; they contain statements indicating that, given access to information (including but not limited to price comparisons), consumers are quite able to judge healthcare offerings properly. In light of the information MTAs provide (including information referred to in all category boxes in Figure 1), and information that the websites say will be collected by savvy consumers from other sources, consumers (the websites say) demonstrate good judgment by selecting offshore care.

Finally, MTA websites mobilize libertarian ideas in making their sales pitch for MTA consumption. For example, in medical travel, one's privacy is respected. This is not only because of legal regulations, adherence to which demonstrates legitimacy, but also, and moreover, because customers have the liberty to seek care without others knowing. One website acknowledged, conspiratorially, 'It is extremely advantageous for certain individuals to go "on vacation" and return home looking refreshed and younger without anyone knowing they received plastic surgery' [16.9].

Elective options can be sought via MTAs without fear of judgement. In addition, there is 'no waiting' and 'less red tape' involved in care procured abroad, such as bariatric surgery (which at home can depend upon proving to gatekeeping authorities that one is a 'good' candidate). 'Elective options' and even procedures 'unavailable in the USA' can be had through offshore sources. A libertarian vision of individual freedom and respect for self-determination is endorsed.

Over- and non-conforming websites

During analysis, a number of websites stood out as different. Two subverted the overarching offer of a 'worry free experience' by focusing on the figure's MTA

Promise strip's categorical themes without actually providing supportive details. One over-emphasized its ability to secure the 'LOWEST cost possible worldwide' [19.1; emphasis in original]. Another, in a bid to present itself as better than the rest, claimed that 'prostitution, child sex trades and underage sex runs rampant in most of the countries that many of these other medical vacation companies send people to' [21.4], drawing excess attention to the issue. Although such amplifications aroused coder suspicion regarding the legitimacy of these MTAs, their over-conformity did substantiate the conceptual model.

Three other websites were categorically different, first in their overall visual emphasis (failing to conform to the blue and white biomedical norm, focusing on touristic vs. medical photos). Second, although qualified for inclusion as comprehensive travel agencies, these MTAs' websites provided little actual information about travel bookings and accommodations. Third, in comparison with the majority of websites, they de-emphasized patient agency.

Further inspection revealed that these MTAs sold mostly wellness and place-based treatments. That is, they sold mostly complementary and alternative medicine – not mostly biomedical travel. For those that sold both, patient-consumers were welcomed generically, rather than differentiated by procedure (specifics were related via drop-down menus in which cardiac surgery might be followed by liposuction). Consumers were thus given the option to align their healthcare needs or desires (many of which would be termed by the dominant biomedical system as 'elective') with biomedicalized, 'legitimate' services.

Discussion

The findings reflect publicly expressed MTA discourse, and the sample was small. Even if representative, because they were frozen in August 2008, the content of these MTA websites may differ from that which might be encountered on live MTA websites today.

Nonetheless, the themes identified fit well with what has been seen in the broader literature on healthcare consumerism and in the emerging ethnographic literature on medical travel. In addition, because of our realistic search strategy, it is likely that the websites 'hit' also would have been among the first MTA websites that patient-consumer searches produced. This plus the fact that two MTA industry members validated our results creates confidence in the research's relevance.

Key findings

Key findings reveal MTA assumptions that potential consumers want 'world class' care (and luxury) for minimal money. Further, they want to be made to feel in control of their health as well as that it is being taken care of by someone else for them, as it would for a VIP.

Conflicting sub-discourses still coherent

The consumer portrayed was not wholly consistent. Some themes coexisted with conflicting ones although, for the potential consumer, conflicts would not be salient because (in addition to being unified in the master tenet of consumerism) each was highlighted in distinct situational contexts, often in separate parts of the websites.

For instance, savvy distrust of medicine at home contrasted with faith in medicine abroad – faith justified by the argument that it is equivalent to medicine at home (e.g., in terms of clinician training, accreditation standards, and so on). Similarly, the ideal of empowered, agentic medical consumerism at home stood in opposition to the hope for facilitated, worry-free, MTA-managed (vs. self-managed) care overseas. Other oppositions included consumer justification of procedures or the medical travel process as 'socially acceptable' and even 'trendy' while seeking to maintain privacy about care procured; the practice of frugality in the face of an expectation for world-class services and VIP treatment; travel to foreign lands without forfeiting access to US-style amenities and US-style medicine; identification with the disenfranchised at home (those denied access to care) but self-construction as members of the global elite through medical travel consumption; the desire for and sense of entitlement to luxury but easy acceptance of low wages and living standards for offshore healthcare workers; and one's serious need for care but concurrent anticipation of an easy recovery allowing for sight-seeing.

MTA marketing appeals to the cultural expectations and ideals for the various subjectivities and self-representations mobilized in its potential customers, each of whom differs depending on (among other things) where he or she is at in the decision-making and travel-undertaking process. The contrapuntal messages following from this within-audience diversity suggests that medical travel involves, for the US-based consumer, a complex, context-dependent act of expressing and forgetting situationally-specific (at home vs. abroad, disenfranchised vs. elite, ill vs. well) self-identities. This process of situational self-reconfiguration and self-representation is cross-culturally common and constant (see de Munck, 1992, 2000; Ewing, 1990). Self-concept shifts, adjusting to the particular as need be (see Holstein and Gubrim 2000). Contradictions inherent in disparate MTA themes are thus non-problematic.

Medical traveller or medical tourist?

MTA website discourse suggests that one situationally preferable identity for potential medical travellers may be that of 'tourist', particularly in order to come to grips with the anticipated experience of recovery. As Sara Ackerman (n.d.) has noted in regard to aesthetic surgery, the post-operative period is often elided by a persuasive and pervasive 'before and after' narrative. This research team observed the same narrative in the website discourse, for aesthetic and non-aesthetic procedures alike. The 'before and after' script reinforces, in its very omission of 'in between', the ideal or the 'speedy recovery'. This is not to say that websites never mentioned a recovery phase – but when they did, the ways in which it is better overseas, not its duration and the debilitation it might entail, were highlighted.

Accordingly, although medical 'travel' more accurately and objectively describes the general process under study (see Sobo 2009; see also Inhorn and Patrizio 2009; Kangas 2010), references to medical 'tourism' may represent a purposive strategy to minimize consumer fears regarding post-surgical debilitation. Thinking of an operation, for instance, as something to be followed (quickly and comfortably) with a trip to the Taj Mahal may in fact feed patient-customer optimism in regard to procedures that always, everywhere, entail risks and recovery costs such as pain, nausea, and exhaustion.

Related to this, the websites' main texts said nothing of the actual risks of particular treatments or procedures. To sell 'worry free' medical travel, this is understandable. Indeed, where risk was addressed it was mostly in terms of how risks were lower and success rates higher offshore, or how the careful vetting done by the MTA mitigated the possibilities (e.g., 'Like any procedures performed locally, procedures done aboard [sic] also carry certain risks. However, by selecting the best accredited hospitals... we minimize this risk substantially' [13.19]). Risk was sometimes mentioned in 'terms and conditions' sections (which two-thirds of the websites had; see Table 1), or in procedure details, but in legalistic language whereby risk was cast as part of the inevitable 'small print' and nothing for the non-paranoid, careful patient-consumer to worry about.

Consumer savvy and patient agency

The US-based MTA market is part of a world where medical consumerism is practised and encouraged (Baer, 2001; Keckley and Eselius, 2009; Lupton, 1997; Sobo, 2001; Williams, 1994). This includes by the government, which offers (among other consumer resources) 'Your guide to choosing quality health care'. This document instructs people to 'make quality health care choices', ominously adding, 'Your good health, and your family's, depends on it'. (Agency for Healthcare Research and Quality 2001, 2). Ensuring access to safe, high-quality care is the consumer's responsibility. The consumer is imagined as having enough agency and self-efficacy – as well as information – to act successfully on this charge.

This simplistic conceptualization of individual responsibility for health deflects attention from structural impediments to such. It also encourages individuals to conceive of the body as a socially significant and self-constructed project – one attained through well-executed healthcare consumerism (cf. Shilling 1993). In a society where consumer rights are celebrated, and getting a 'good deal' or added value is something to be proud of, the patient's (or potential patient's) self-esteem and the (real or imagined) esteem in which others hold him or her can be enhanced through actively and wisely self-managing care – as through smartly booking medical travel.

For this reason, most MTA websites highlight savvy consumerism and patient agency. They celebrate the client who takes charge of his or her care through medical travel. The wise medical consumer or 'Wisdom' narrative, described in regard to elective surgery seekers and seen in discourse on indicated surgeries by proxy decision-makers (Sobo 2001, 2005), is replicated in MTA website content – albeit in a co-conspiratorial way that emphasizes not only wisdom but also know-how and confidence ('savvy').

Variation

The emphasis on patient agency within the 'savvy consumer' category did differ between websites that sold biomedicine mainly and those that sold mainly complementary and alternative medicine (CAM), such as Ayurvedic or spa treatment. Biomedically-oriented sites highlighted agency while CAM websites did not – perhaps because increased patient agency already exists among those opting for CAM.

We interpret the overt emphasis on patient agency in biomedically-oriented sites as reflecting biomedical patient-consumer demand for it (see also Cohen 2008, 226). The emphasis may also be related to class re-identification strategies promoted. Medical travellers seeking biomedical treatment overseas may be disproportionately representative of the working poor, who have limited access to affordable care at home. The idea of personal agency may tie in for them with the 'American Dream' of claiming a place at the top of the social structure. It also may be a way to claim more control in a political economy that, despite all-American libertarian rhetoric, puts full self-determination beyond many people's reach.

World-class care for the global elite

In many ways the websites provide a critique of the US healthcare delivery model – a critique that, if heeded by US-based healthcare organizations, might prove constructive. But it cannot offset the fact that a new 'world class' of clinical care has emerged, and although it is 'Western' and 'cutting edge', it is not synonymous with 'American'. New processes and procedures increasingly have transnational origins (*Economist* 2008b; Inhorn and Birenbaum-Carmeli 2008, 180). Physical healthcare spaces dedicated to medical travel have been observed not as 'little Americas' but rather generic transnational spaces, like international airport hotels (Whittaker 2008, 284).

The eclipse of 'American' by 'world-class' medical care reflects globalizations' prioritization of transnational connections over national boundaries (Hannerz 1996). It is supported by MTA website discourse overshadowing nationalism by highlighting as needed the existence of a global elite partaking 'world class' services – a group that MTA customers would be a part of.

Conclusion

Holstein and Gubrium (2000, 95) follow Foucault and Hughes to argue that particular self-constructions are 'incited' by the institutional or organizational sites that individuals engage with. Accordingly, while MTA website messages must *have* cultural appeal or resonate with pre-existing cultural desires and self-concepts if they are to turn a profit, they also *make* cultural appeals in the discursive resources they offer, providing 'the conditions of possibility' and supplying 'the mode of production for putting into effect our identities as part of accomplishing matters of ongoing [immediate] interest' (Holstein and Gubrium 2000, 95). In this way, MTAs may not only catalogue but also help create or reinforce particular consumer self-constructions. As such, they may play an important catalysing role in healthcare consumerism's evolution and therefore in the ongoing evolution of healthcare per se.

Prominent MTA website themes suggest – and may help ensure through their discursive influence – that the US medical travel consumer wants 'world-class' care at a low financial cost. He or she also wants to be a particular type of person – a person ahead of the trends – a person of high station who has a right to luxury, and to control what happens, while depending on others to carry out directions on his or her behalf. Cultural expectations and ideals representing 'American' aspirations underwrite the appeal of particular self-perceptions that can be situationally actualized or incited for US patient-consumers considering medical travel.

Acknowledgements

A portion of this work was funded by a 'faculty fellowship' grant from the Ethics Center in Science and Technology. Ethics approval was unnecessary due to the public nature of the data. No conflicts of interest existed. Diane Boyd, President of the medical travel agency Affordable World Care, provided expert feedback over the course of the study. Erik Cohen and Beth Kangas kindly provided early guidance and reading suggestions, as did later anonymous reviewers, and Kent Sandstrom, to whom the authors owe great thanks. The article's focus on self-contradictions was driven in part by self-contradicting (and self-revealing) responses to preliminary findings presented in the University of California Berkeley/University of California San Francisco Medical Anthropology and History of Health Sciences Colloquium series (22 April 2009). The authors alone remain responsible for the article's content.

Notes

1. In addition to helping patients, offshore providers can positively affect the communities where they are situated. In some host countries, medical travel income may be reinvested in the national health infrastructure (Siegel 2007). Hospitals catering to medical travellers employ local residents. Job creation fuelled by the medical travel boom may even lead more supply-zone residents to seek medical training, adding to local knowledge and perhaps increasing the sustainability of programmes serving the local poor as well. Moreover, as medical travel fuels healthcare's growth in home countries, nurses, doctors, and other healthcare specialists who previously emigrated to places like the USA or UK may return home – or stay home to start. Trinidad and India, for example, have seen doctors return (*Economist*, 2008b). Costs, too, may be entailed. For instance, the globalized demand for gestational surrogates may exploit poor women, putting them at risk for complications during impregnation, gestation, and childbirth (e.g., when caesarean sections are undertaken to make the birth convenient for the intended legal parents) (Kumar 2008). Communities can suffer as healthcare resources are diverted to serve rich foreign nationals. However, as *The Economist* has noted, 'state-run health bureaucracies in developing countries... neglected the poor long before medical tourists arrived' (*Economist* 2008a). Indeed, rather than simply creating new inequities, medical travel may more commonly serve to recreate existing class, gender, and race/nationality-based inequities.
2. This was not a starting point for the project but rather a point of arrival for us.
3. Many disciplines other than anthropology use ethnographic methods and many have understood them differently from how anthropologists might. The label here is not reflective of a traditional anthropological understanding of the meaning of ethnography per se. Rather, it reveals an appreciation of the iterative approach that anthropologists generally take toward ethnographic data, which it would apply to media sources. The method is thereby useful for examining mediated practices and processes that local- or geographically-defined boundaries fail to ring-fence.

References

Ackerman, S. n.d. Plastic paradise: Transforming bodies and selves in Costa Rica's cosmetic surgery tourism industry. Pre-publication version dated 5 May 2009. This paper has since been published in *Medical Anthropology* 29, no. 4.

Agency for Healthcare Research and Quality. 2001. Your guide to choosing quality health care. AHRQ Publication No. 99-0012. Rockville, MD: Agency for Healthcare Research and Quality.

Altheide, D.L. 1987. Ethnographic content analysis. *Qualitative Sociology* 10, no. 1: 65–77.

Altheide, D.L. 2000. Identity and the definition of the situation in a mass-mediated context. *Symbolic Interaction* 23, no. 1: 1–27.

Anonymous. 2006. Medical tourism, Asia's growth industry: Hotelmarketing.com.

Baer, H.A. 2001. *Biomedicine and alternative healing systems in America: Issues of class, race, ethnicity, and gender.* Madison: University of Wisconsin Press.

Bookman, M.Z., and K.R. Bookman. 2007. *Medical tourism in developing countries.* New York: Palgrave Macmillan.

Bramstedt, K., and J. Xu. 2007. Checklist: Passport, plane ticket, organ transplant. *American Journal of Transplantation* 7: 1698–701.

Burns, E. 2008. U.S. search engine rankings. December 2007: SearchEngineWatch.com.

Carrol, J. 2007. Long-distance medicine: U.S. businesses are looking overseas for a way to keep employee health-care costs down. *American Way* 56–57.

Cohen, E. 2008. Medical tourism in Thailand. In *Explorations in Thai tourism: Collected case studies,* ed. E. Cohen, 225–55. Bingley: Emerald Group.

de Munck, V. 1992. The fallacy of the misplaced self: Gender relations and the construction of multiple selves among Sri Lankan Muslims. *Ethos,* 20, no. 2: 167–90.

de Munck, V. 2000. *Culture, self, and meaning.* Long Grove, IL: Waveland Press.

Economist. 2008a. Leaders: Importing competition; Globalisation and health. *The Economist* 388: 8593.

Economist. 2008b. Operating profit; Globalisation and health care. *The Economist,* 388: 8593.

Ewing, K.P. 1990. The illusion of wholeness: 'Culture,' 'self,' and the experience of inconsistency. *Ethos* 18, no. 3: 251–78.

Garcia, A.C., A.I. Standlee, J. Bechkof, and Y. Cui. 2009. Ethnographic approaches to the internet and computer-mediated communication. *Journal of Contemporary Ethnography* 38, no. 1: 52–84.

Glaser, B.G., and A. Strauss. 1967. *The discovery of grounded theory: Strategies for qualitative research.* New York: Aldine de Gruyter.

Gunasekera, V., E. Ernst, and D.G. Ezra. 2008. Systematic Internet-based review of complementary and alternative medicine for glaucoma. *Ophthamology* 115: 435–9.

Hannerz, U. 1996. *Transnational connections: Culture, people, places.* New York: Routledge.

Higgins, L.A. 2007. Medical tourism takes off, but not without debate. *Managed Care* 16, no. 4: 45–47.

Hill, J. 2005. Finding culture in narrative. In *Finding culture in talk: A collection of methods,* ed. N. Quinn, 157–202. New York: Palgrave Macmillan.

Holstein, J.A., and J.F. Gubrium. 2000. *The self we live by: Narrative identity in a postmodern world.* New York: Oxford University Press.

Inhorn, M., and P. Patrizio. 2009. Rethinking reproductive 'tourism' as reproductive 'exile'. *Fertility and Sterility* 29, no. 3: 904–6.

Inhorn, M.C., and D. Birenbaum-Carmeli. 2008. Assisted reproductive technologies and culture change. *Annual Reviews in Anthropology* 37: 177–96.

Kangas, B. 2002. Therapeutic itineraries in a global world: Yemenis and their search for biomedical treatment abroad. *Medical Anthropology* 21, no. 1: 35–78.

Kangas, B. 2007. Hope from abroad in the international medical travel of Yemeni patients. *Anthropology and Medicine* 14, no. 3: 293–305.

Kangas, B. 2010. Travelling for medical care in a global world. *Medical Anthropology* 29, no. 4: 344–62.

Keckley, P.H., and L.L. Eselius. 2009. *2009 survey of health care consumers key findings, strategic implications.* Washington, DC: Deloitte Center for Health Solutions, Deloitte Development LLC.

Keckley, P.H., and H.R. Underwood. 2008. *Medical tourism: Consumers in search of value.* Washington, DC: Deloitte Center for Health Solutions.

Kumar, P. 2008. Indian surrogacy: Blessing, business or both? *Neem Magazine* 1, no. 4, http://www.neemmagazine.com/culture63

Lupton, D. 1997. Consumerism, reflexivity and the medical encounter. *Social Science and Medicine* 45: 373–81.

Milstein, A., and M. Smith. 2006. America's new refugees – Seeking affordable surgery offshore. *New England Journal of Medicine* 355, no. 16: 1637–40.

Norris, M.L., K.M. Boydell, L. Pinhas, and D.K. Katzman. 2006. Ana and the internet: A review of pro-anorexia websites. *International Journal of Eating Disorders* 39, no. 6: 443–7.

Quinn, N. 2005. How to reconstruct schemas people share, from what they say. In *Finding culture in talk: A collection of methods*, ed. N. Quinn, 35–81. New York: Palgrave Macmillan.

Ryan, G.W., and H.R. Bernard. 2003. Techniques to identify themes. *Field Methods* 15, no. 1: 85–109.

Salinger, S., L. Plonka, and L. Prechelt. 2008. A coding scheme development methodology using grounded theory for qualitative analysis of pair programming. *Human Technology* 4, no. 1: 9–25.

Scheper-Hughes, N. 2002. The ends of the body: Commodity fetishism and the global traffic in organs. *SAIS Review* XXII, no. 1: 61–80.

Shilling, C. 1993. *The body and social theory*. London: Sage.

Siegel, J. 2007. Hadassah uses internet to attract foreign surgical patients. *Jerusalem Post* p. 5.

Sobo, E.J. 2001. Rationalization of medical risk through talk of trust: An exploration of elective eye surgery narratives. *Anthropology and Medicine* 8, no. 2/3: 265–78.

Sobo, E.J. 2005. Parents' perceptions of pediatric day surgery risks: Unforeseeable complications, or avoidable mistakes? *Social Science and Medicine* 60, no. 10: 2341–50.

Sobo, E.J. 2009. Medical travel: What it means and why it matters. *Medical Anthropology* 29, no. 1: 326–35.

Speier, A. 2008. IVF vacation: Providing 'modern' fertility treatments at lower costs. *Annual Meeting of the American Anthropological Association*. San Francisco.

Strauss, A., and J. Corbin. 1998. *Basics of qualitative research: Techniques and procedures for developing grounded theory*. Thousand Oaks, CA: Sage.

Van Esch, S.C.M., M.C. Cornel, and F.J. Snoek. 2006. Type 2 diabetes and inheritance: What information do diabetes organizations provide on the Internet? *Diabetic Medicine* 23: 1233–8.

Whittaker, A. 2008. Pleasure and pain: Medical travel in Asia. *Global Public Health* 3, no. 3: 271–290.

Williams, B. 1994. Patient satisfaction: A valid concept? *Social Science and Medicine* 38: 509–16.

AFTERWORD

Historical reflections on medical travel

George Weisz

Department of Social Studies of Medicine, McGill University, Montréal, Canada

The terms 'medical tourism' and 'health tourism' cover many phenomena. Individuals able to afford the costs have frequently traveled great distances to consult with healers considered especially competent in their field. A reputation for expertise has, for the past century, been linked to technological capacity and those who can do so may prefer to travel to places such as the Mayo Clinic rather than relying on technology and expertise available locally. In Canada, there is something like a tradition that provincial Premiers with serious illnesses travel to the United States for their medical care. This is always controversial since Premiers are supposedly responsible for the quality of provincial health-care systems; if they don't trust these institutions why should the rest of us? But despite occasional bursts of outrage, most Canadians understand the desire to obtain the best possible medical care even if it means traveling outside the country. What is unusual about the newest sort of 'health tourism' discussed in several papers in this issue is that technology and excellence are only some of the attracting features. Relatively low costs, desire to avoid waiting lists, access to procedures or facilities unavailable and possibly illegal at home, are often determining factors in individual decisions to travel for health care. One factor that is less than central is place. It just happens that the Mayo Clinic is in Rochester Minnesota, or the Cleveland Clinic is in Cleveland Ohio, or that the institutions discussed in these pages are located where they are. Location of course is not irrelevant. Not every locale can bring together the expertise, technology, capital, easy access and relative lack of political violence that turns a city into a medical destination. But there is nothing about these places that is intrinsically healthy or good for you. In many ways, 'tourism' is a catchy misnomer that simply means traveling long distances for medical care not dissimilar to what is available at home. While this phenomenon has relevance for medical care and global health and for the ways social scientists study them, such practices can best be seen as yet another example of the expanding global economy, another form of 'offshoring' goods and services, whose consequences have yet to be fully understood. It in no way diminishes the significance of this phenomenon to note that its application to health care is too recent for historians to have much in the way of a contribution to make to its discussion.

There is, however, another form of medical tourism about which historians can say a good deal. It involves the close relationship between medical care and what is conventionally understood as 'tourism', which is closely tied to specific locations. That is to say, the therapy and the pleasures of tourism are inextricably linked and are intimately associated with specific places considered especially 'healthy' and, not inconsequentially, pleasant and attractive: the hilltop stations of colonial India; mountain tuberculosis sanatoria; and among the earliest examples, mineral waters spas. Many papers in this issue are about these latter institutions, which have received considerable attention from scholars, at least in part because of their rich hybrid character. Spas provided specific forms of therapy that were for many centuries part of mainstream medicine; here I need to distinguish mineral waters from other forms of hydrotherapy, like Vincent Priessnitz's famous cold water system that was unquestionably 'alternative' rather than mainstream (Marland and Adams 2009). True mineral waters were very much connected with place and were frequently thought to lose their therapeutic powers if they were moved to another location, so people had to travel to them. In order to attract clients from afar to submit to sometimes unpleasant regimens and to keep them and accompanying families from running off to more interesting places, spas (or thermal stations as they are frequently called in France) have also been places of tourist leisure where walks, socializing, music, dance, theatre and even gambling became part of the healing experience. Movement has not been all in one direction. Jill Steward (2000) has suggested that some Austro-Hungarian spas began as resorts and only later added medicinal use of waters to their offerings because this attracted more tourists. The balance between the two functions varies significantly from one spa and one era to the next. In some cases I can say definitively that one or the other dominates. In many other cases, they coexist in permanent symbiosis or tension. In addition to being places of therapy, healing and pleasure, spas have also constituted social spaces in which individuals and social classes enact elaborate social rituals that have fascinated novelists and filmmakers. To some degree they reproduce normative social arrangements and distinctions, albeit in a uniquely intense and small-scale setting. At the same time they can be liminal spaces where normal rules of social life are relaxed; where nobility and middle class individuals can mingle; where, according to novelists and filmmakers, love affairs, licit and illicit, are possible and even incest seems like innocent fun (*Le Souffle au Coeur* by Louis Malle). They can serve as metaphors for a way of life, indeed a civilization, that is about to disappear (*Badenheim 1939*, by Aaron Applefeld).

The social aspects of the spa experience are so compelling that they have tended to overshadow discussion of their medical functions. The papers in this issue are a welcome exception to this tendency and remind us that spas have been, in the first instance, places of healing. The term itself is more complex than one might think. There is, first of all, the 'medical' as it has come to be understood: for example, physicians prescribing a growing variety of procedures based on waters seen as far more potent than normal tap water but gentler and more natural than most other therapies; other physicians supervising a therapeutic process that can have unexpected and expected side effects, such as fevers (thermal crises) that are thought to be beneficial but must be closely monitored. France certainly provides the most dramatic example of this sort of medicalized thermalism, largely due to the fact that responsibility for the nations' spas fell to the premier institution of medical research in nineteenth-century France, the Paris Academy of Medicine. But medical practitioners, in France as elsewhere, have frequently been ambivalent or even skeptical about the powers or water and in some countries – Germany is perhaps the prime example, but also Brazil as M.M. Quintela's paper in this issue indicates (Quintela 2011) – mineral waters have been seen as a form of alternative or complementary medicine, a natural substitute for the practices of conventional medicine. Where alternative medicines are widely tolerated by health authorities, as is the case in Germany, water cures are reimbursed by the health insurance system. In the United States where spas were for the most part almost purely commercial establishments, they have been seen mainly as a form of charlatanism. (During the 1920s and 30s, influenced by European models, Americans created medicalized spas, like those of Saratoga Springs, but the boom did not last long.) As forms of either orthodox or alternative healing, mineral water spas usually dealt with chronic illnesses of one sort or another and the goal was less often to cure than to alleviate symptoms and bring relief, which might well be temporary. Hence repeated trips to the spa were required.

Finally, and less frequently noted by scholars of the modern period – although this is a mainstay of scholarship of the ancient world (Galliou 2006) – waters could be a source of religious-based healing. The waters of Monchique were long a setting of religious healing as Cristiana Bastos shows in this issue (Bastos 2011). The spas of Pyrmont were originally devoted to miraculous healing before becoming centers of naturalistic water cures (Lempa 2008). To this day, the waters of Lourdes are thought to contain special spiritual properties that can produce miraculous cures. The Catholic hierarchy has been ambivalent about such miraculous cures and long ago set up an office to distinguish the small number of truly miraculous cures from fallacious claims (Szabo 2002). One cannot help thinking that the powers of even naturalistically understood cures rest to some extent on the primordial qualities popularly attributed to water generally and especially those waters whose sources lies deep under the earth's surface. The ritualistic regularity of spa life represents yet another link to its religious past.

Spas of course were not just places of healing. They were tourist destinations and social spaces. As tourist destinations they had to develop non-therapeutic infrastructures – railway lines, hotels, parks, casinos, which frequently financed therapeutic activities. These amenities were not just necessary to attract curists and the family and friends who might accompany them; they were an integral part of the cure. Even in France where water cures were seen as form of natural chemotherapy, no one doubted that leisure, relaxation, fresh air, and general escape from urban stress to natural rural beauty all intervened to intensify the therapeutic effects of waters. In other locales these aspects might be seen as the essential elements of the curing process with waters playing a secondary role. The relationship between tourist leisure and therapy was not without conflicts. Spa doctors frequently mistrusted the commercial propensities of proprietors and doubted their commitment to medicalized therapy. They complained bitterly about the heavy meals frequently served in expensive spa hotels. Above all, they feared becoming mere tourist sites. Nonetheless, doctors and entrepreneurs were inextricably bound together and, by the early twentieth century, spas were a recognized if highly specialized part of local tourist industries and were organized to maximize resources and efficiency in an increasingly competitive market. This meant, in particular, new and more sophisticated forms of advertising but it also involved expanding leisure and tourist services as well as technologies for dispensing water cures. Aside from modernizing medical facilities, it was necessary to deliver healing waters in new ways, via vapors, pulverization, showers, mud baths or through previously ignored orifices. It might also mean expanding health activities beyond waters to include procedures such as massage and physiotherapy. In an intensely competitive environment, in which spas battled one another to attract clients, success in combining the latest medical innovations with the latest tourist amenities might mean the difference between institutional success and failure.

There have been interesting efforts to analyze the specific role that spa therapy played in the expansion of the tourist industry. It has been suggested that vacationing for the purposes of health was one of the first socially acceptable forms of leisure for the bourgeoisie, since its essential purpose – promoting health and vigor – was valued by the rising middle classes. It thus made leisure compatible with a bourgeois work ethic (Mackaman 1998). While such theories are stimulating, historians simply do not know enough about the early development of tourism to attribute so much importance to the role of health maintenance. It has been postulated that spas served other roles as well. In his book on French colonial spas, Eric Jennings (2006) speculates that local watering holes provided colonists with a dose of the French metropolis that was missing from the usual places of colonial social interaction and that periodic visits to the spas of France, notably Vichy, allowed officials and colonists from throughout the Empire to mingle and develop a common identity. Again, such ideas are plausible and deserve consideration, but scholars need to know far more about actual social interactions in such places in order to do more than speculate. Lauren LaFauci has taken a major step in this direction in her essay in this issue. Here she presents a dense and well-documented argument about the role of southern spas in developing southern identity and actually helping to consolidate support for slavery (LaFauci 2011). In a rather different vein, Steward (2002) has described how spas in the Austro-Hungarian Empire fostered local identities among ethnic groups such as Magyars, Poles and the like. This was not just a case of people being more comfortable with their own kind. Nationalisms might be exploited to attract groups to specific spas in spite of powerful attractions drawing them to more cosmopolitan locations.

There is a general view that spas in the eighteenth century were largely aristocratic destinations. This is somewhat oversimplified because it focuses on a handful of fashionable towns, such as Bath and Baden Baden, and ignores the large number of thermal sources with more modest ambitions and facilities. French spas of the early modern period were, in Laurence Brockliss's account, spartan places (Brockliss 1990). But the few fashionable spas undoubtedly influenced popular stereotypes surrounding the spa experience. A corollary of this view is that spas with a strong aristocratic flavor became more middle class as the nineteenth century progressed. This was certainly likely as the middle classes expanded and more people were able to pay the considerable costs of the spa cure. But as a number of studies remind us, there was always considerable diversity among spa guests. One historian sees the German spa of the later eighteenth century as a space of bourgeois-noble interaction that helped create enlightenment culture (Kuhnert 1984). And such diversity increased over time. A historian of American spas sees them as spaces where national integration took place on a limited scale during the latter decades of the nineteenth century (Chambers 2002). Spas also divided social classes. David Blackbourn (2002) has emphasized the elitist character of certain fashionable European spas catering to an international elite that traveled from one fashionable spa to another. Steward (2002) suggests that such behavior repelled the middle of classes of Hapsburg Austria who preferred the simpler more regimen-based resorts such as Carlsbad or Gräfenberg.

If diversity characterized spas in their balance among social classes or emphasis on therapy as opposed to leisure, the same may be said about their success in attracting clients. In the US, spas were always fairly marginal institutions because, as suggested here, they were linked by the medical profession to charlatanism. But Britain had a vibrant spa industry in the eighteenth century, boasting world famous institutions like those of Bath, which gradually lost their popularity and luster in the second half of the nineteenth century. To explain this decline by appealing to changing fashions is a form of tautology (they became less popular because they became less popular) and ignores the fact that the appeal of continental spas increased dramatically during the period of British decline. To one analyst, it was the capitalist structure of the industries in the different countries that best explains their diverging histories. While English spas were primarily private sector speculations, those of Germany were part of a system of state-managed capitalism that produced resource-rich, innovative and attractive resorts (Bacon 1997). Much the same can be said of French spas that also expanded dramatically during this period with the help of significant state (national and local) funding and regulation. Whether this explanation is correct or not, it is always nice to be reminded that private enterprise has its limitations and state intervention its uses.

However, resources and facilities tell only part of the story. There is also the science of mineral waters, which has been surprisingly understudied. Explaining the way waters operated therapeutically has traditionally been the province of medical science. For much of the nineteenth and twentieth centuries, efficacy or lack thereof have been perceived as matters of empirical fact (see Weisz 2001). The task of science was to explain how these waters actually worked. Chemistry was the chief instrument in performing this task. Analyzing chemical composition (a sophisticated scientific activity in itself) served as a basis for classifying waters and suggested theories of physiological mechanism. Such theories changed regularly as new scientific tools made new entities (such as radiation) visible but the goal of explaining mechanisms remained primary. In France, a second and linked goal was to use knowledge of mechanisms to permit increasingly specialized use of waters for specific ailments in a manner that approximated the most modern therapeutics. While it was understood that the rest, relaxation, and the beauty of the countryside had a role to play in therapy, it was the chemical composition of the waters that normalized human physiology. One could represent the encounter as one between two complex liquids with one adding to or drawing from the other specific elements. In the words of the second professor of hydrology at the Paris Faculty of Medicine, Maurice Chiray, '[m]ineral waters are, like the liquids of the organism, a complex electrolic milieu, and the infinitely small [elements] of one can act on the infinitely small [elements] of the other, either by way of the exchanges of certain elements, or by way of the addition of others which the humors are partially or totally lacking' (Chiray 1938). As the century progressed, interpretations centering on the nervous system as the regulator of physiological terrain became more common. By the early twentieth century, the French were doing more than speculating. A network of university chairs devoted to thermalism was created and financed by the waters industry and produced a growing literature on the physical effects of waters. Little of this research was clinical. Not only was efficacy presumed, but clinical research had little status in the early twentieth century. The hallmark of science was laboratory experimentation and French university laboratories went energetically about the business of testing the effects of different waters on animals or isolated organs. Such work could say little about clinical efficacy but it produced a large literature demonstrating that waters produced physiological effects. It was a leap but not a huge one to attribute therapeutic effects to such physiological effects. By the 1940s, the network of academic chairs and laboratories had become so visible and had produced a large enough body of scientific literature that few questioned thermalism's place in French medicine or its reimbursement by the social insurance system that was introduced following the Second World War.

However, this golden age did not last. In the first instance, medical science provided a host of therapies that worked more quickly and consistently (although not necessarily more cheaply) than did mineral waters. In the second, health insurance systems quickly found themselves in financial trouble. It was tempting to try to save money by cutting back on reimbursement of services that appeared increasingly old-fashioned. Finally, definitions of scientific validity changed. Even before the 'evidence-based medicine' movement turned such ideas into scientific orthodoxy, there was increasing disenchantment with a purely experimental approach that justified therapies by appealing to presumed underlying physiological mechanisms corrected by waters. The demand here, as throughout medicine, was for proof of therapeutic efficacy via double-blind, randomized clinical trials, sufficiently numerous to permit meta-analysis. This was a difficult jump for spa industries to make, even in places such as France and Portugal where they were highly medicalized. Some spas thus jumped into the alternative medicine camp, which did not at that time demand randomized clinical trials to demonstrate efficacy. One could even abandon water and find new therapeutic modalities, although few institutions that changed their orientation displayed the inspired creativity of the Ayurvedic spa described by Harish Naraindas in this issue (Naraindas 2011). Another option was to move into the 'wellness' business and provide essentially healthy people with services that make them feel good or better, everything from massages, to perfumed baths to facials. This strategy had the advantage of not requiring the total abandonment of medicalized waters but merely adding new services to existing water treatments. As Cristiana Bastos and Amy Speier demonstrate in this issue, such hybrid institutions can work fairly well, quite possibly because they do – in a more expansive and targeted way – something that successful spas have always done: add pleasure and well-being to an essentially medical enterprise (Bastos 2011, Speier 2011).

French spas have also experimented with the provision of such services in an effort to deal with declining interest and funding. Those of the Jura (in the mountainous east of the country) now distinguish between two types of clients. In 2002, those taking traditional thermal cures accounted for about 25% of the economic benefits of the industry and were usually over 60 years of age, excepting those visiting several spas that specialize in children; such cures lasted the canonic 21 days. In addition, about 10% of revenues was due to a much larger group of visitors seeking a return to form (*remise en form*) during stays lasting about 6 days (which explains why they generated less revenue) and who were characteristically between 40 and 60 years of age.[1] A national study in 2002 found that 95% of all days spent in spas were devoted to medical cures while 5% were devoted to *remise en form*.[2]

If movement toward this wellness orientation continues to occur at the local level, and even famous spas like Aix-les-Bains push this aggressively in their online advertising, it is largely absent from political and medical discourse. In fact, most such rhetoric has to do with adapting mineral waters to new criteria of evidence-based research. The impetus, it is true, has come from the French government, which gave notice in 2000 that it would not continue to reimburse cures unless the industry was able to justify not just the efficacy of its practices, but the efficacy and economic advantages over other forms of therapy. By 2002, an accord had been signed to this effect and the spa industry – as it had in the 1920s and 1930s – intervened, financially allocating over a million euros annually for research. A new research organization AFRETH (Association Française pour la Recherche Thermale) was set up in 2005 and by the end of 2009, had financed 23 research projects, studying the effects of waters on such varied conditions as thrombosis, otitis, anxiety and obesity.[3] A recent clinical trial has apparently demonstrated that water cures are significantly more effective than a standard anxiolytic, paroxetine, for reducing the symptoms of anxiety (Dubois et al. 2008). Thermal-station and university laboratories have also engaged in research using local funds. Spending a little over €1,000,000 annually on such research hardly puts AFRETH in the same league as the French INSERM, let alone the National Institutes of Health. But as a symbol of willingness to adapt to new scientific and political imperatives, it says much about the French determination to keep mineral waters if not in the mainstream then at least within the margins of contemporary biomedicine.

Notes

1. Le Tourisme thermale, http://www.cdt-jura.fr/upload/paragraphes/1084183199.PDF (accessed June 9 2010).
2. Aspects économiques du thermalisme français, Slide 5.1. http://portaildoc.oieau.fr/entrepotsOAI/OIEAU/44/223202/223202_doc.pdf (uploaded June 9 2010).
3. http://www.afreth.org/docprojet/suivi.htm (uploaded June 10 2010).

References

Bacon, W. 1997. The rise of the German and the demise of the English spa industry: A critical analysis of business success and failure. *Leisure Studies* 16: 173–87.

Bastos, Cristiana. 2011. From sulphur to perfume: Spa and SPA at Monchique, Algarve. *Anthropology and Medicine* 18, no. 1: 37–53.

Blackbourn, D. 2002. Fashionable spa towns in nineteenth-century Europe. In *Water, leisure, and culture: European historical perspectives*, ed. Susan C. Anderson and Bruce H. Tabb, 9–21. Oxford, New York: Berg.

Brockliss, L.W.B. 1990. The development of the spa in seventeenth-century France in the medical history of waters and spas. *Medical History. Supplement* 10: 23–47.

Chambers, Thomas A. 2002. *Drinking the waters: Creating an American leisure class at nineteenth-century mineral springs*. Washington and London: Smithsonian Institution Press.

Chiray, Maurice. 1938. Leçon d'ouverture: Chaire d'hydrologie thérapeutique et de climatologie. *La Presse médicale* 46: 253.

Dubois, O., R. Salamon, M. Poirier, and J. Olié. 2008. Le thermalisme psychiatrique dans les troubles anxieux; crenotherapy in anxiety disorder. *Annales Médico-Psychologiques* 166: 109–14.

Galliou, Patrick. 2006. Water, water everywhere…water, ailing bodies and the gods in Roman Gaul and Britain. In *Spas in Britain and in France in the eighteenth and nineteenth centuries*, ed. Annick Cossic and Patrick Galliou, 9–21. Cambridge: Cambridge Scholars Press.

Jennings, Eric T. 2006. *Curing the colonizers: hydrotherapy, climatology, and French colonial spas*. Durham and London: Duke University Press.

Kuhnert, Reinhold P. 1984. Urbanitat auf dem Lande. Badereisen nach Pyrmont im 18. Jahrhundert. *Veroffentlichungen des Max-PlanckInstituts für Geschichte* 77. Gottingen, Vandenhoeck & Ruprecht.

LaFauci, Lauren E. 2011. Taking the (southern) waters: Science, slavery, and nationalism at the antebellum Virginia Springs. *Anthropology and Medicine* 18, no. 1: 7–22.

Lempa, Heike. 2008. The spa: Emotional economy and social classes in nineteenth-century Pyrmont. *Central European History* 35, no. 1: 37–73.

Mackaman, Douglas Peter. 1998. *Leisure settings: Bourgeois culture, medicine and the spa in modern France*. Chicago and London: University of Chicago Press.

Marland, Hilary, and Jane Adams. 2009. Hydropathy at home: The water cure and domestic healing in mid-nineteenth-century Britain. *Bulletin of the History of Medicine* 83: 499–529.

Naraindas, Harish. 2011. Of relics, body parts and laser beams: The German Heilpraktiker and his Ayurvedic Spa. *Anthropology and Medicine* 18, no. 1: 67–86.

Quintela, Maria Manuel. 2011. Seeking 'energy' vs. pain relief in spas in Brazil (Caldas da Imperatriz) and Portugal (Termas da Sulfúrea). *Anthropology and Medicine* 18, no. 1: 23–35.

Speier, Amy. 2011. Health tourism in a Czech spa. *Anthropology and Medicine* 18, no. 1: 55–66.

Steward, Jill. 2000. The spa towns of the Austro-Hungarian Empire and the growth of tourist culture, 1860-1914. In *New directions in urban history: Aspects of European art, health, tourism and leisure since the enlightenment*, ed. Peter Borsay, Günther Hirschfelder and Ruth-E. Mohrmann, 87–125. Munster: Waxmann Verlag.

Steward, J. 2002. The culture of water cure in nineteenth-century Austria, 1800–1914. In *Water, leisure and culture: European historical perspectives*, ed. S.C. Anderson and B.H. Tabb, 23–35. Oxford, New York: Berg.

Szabo, Jason. 2002. Seeing is believing? The form and substance of French medical debates over Lourdes. *Bulletin of the History of Medicine* 76, no. 2: 199–230.

Weisz, George. 2001. Spas, mineral waters and hydrological science in twentieth-century France. *Isis* 92: 451–83.

Index

Printed and bound by CPI Group (UK) Ltd, Croydon, CR0 4YY

24/10/2024

01778293-0018